Praise for *Attacking M...*

"As an entrepreneur and lifelong friend ... commitment and vision in striving to conquer this chronic disease. . . . ... has once again welded his medical expertise and business acumen to create a dynamic undertaking for the wellness of mankind. I urge all business leaders of the community with a deep conviction of caregiving to support the ultimate caregiver in his quest for healthcare excellence for all those affected by autoimmune diseases." — JOE A. CHAMBLISS, CHAIRMAN, THE CHAMBLISS GROUP, FORT LAUDERDALE, FLORIDA

". . . illustrates the typically American approach to a medical problem: personal entrepreneurship, exemplified by private non-profit volunteer health agencies. These, such as the American Cancer Society, American Heart Association, or the smaller Cystic Fibrosis Foundation and others, have promoted research and made major inroads in many diseases, actually leading to cure for some, such as choriocarcinoma. I recommend this book for anyone who wants to join the fight." — JAMES A. PITTMAN, JR., M.D., DEAN OF MEDICINE EMERITUS AND DISTINGUISHED PROFESSOR, UNIVERSITY OF ALABAMA AT BIRMINGHAM (UAB)

". . . an excellent read for all individuals impacted by myasthenia gravis and other chronic diseases. Relying on a keen intellect, inner strength, clarity of vision, and the power of positive thinking, Dr. Henderson tells the story of his personal battle with MG. In so doing, he provides guidelines for patients and caregivers confronted with the emotional and physical challenges of chronic disease. The book also emphasizes the importance of supporting cutting-edge research in immune-mediated diseases. This is necessary for unraveling the mysteries of MG and other autoimmune diseases and for laying a foundation for the development of safer and more efficacious treatment strategies."— ARNOLD I. LEVINSON, M.D., SPECIALIST IN DIAGNOSIS, TREATMENT, AND RESEARCH OF IMMUNE-MEDIATED DISEASE, PROFESSOR OF MEDICINE AND NEUROLOGY, UNIVERSITY OF PENNSYLVANIA SCHOOL OF MEDICINE

"How does one, whose body has only one gear, *overdrive*, survive the free fall from the mountaintop of ultimate achievement and maxed-out motivation to the rock-bottom MG valley of the weakest of the weak? Dr. Ron Henderson's book is the best *role model road map* toward *the land of beginning again* that a chronic disease patient could ever follow." — JAMES D. MOEBES, PH.D., SENIOR MINISTER, MOUNTAIN BROOK BAPTIST CHURCH, BIRMINGHAM, ALABAMA

". . . an inspirational and informative book which all chronic disease patients, their families, and physicians should read and reread. Written by my college and medical school classmate, fellow obstetrician-gynecologist, and lifelong friend, this book reflects Ron's humanitarianism, intellect, and courage against adversity. Some books need to be written, and this is [one] — penned by a man whose life has honored our profession." — SAM ENGELHARDT III, M.D., MEDICAL DIRECTOR, JULIA TUTWILER PRISON FOR WOMEN, WETUMPKA, ALABAMA

"As a practicing rheumatologist, I recommend this book to patients and caregivers alike; a superb discussion of the requisite interactions required for successful management of chronic care. As a laboratory researcher, I agree . . . [on] the need for basic research . . . [of] the mechanisms of . . . autoimmune diseases like MG. [And] . . . I agree . . . that the shared pathophysiology of autoimmune disease provides a unique forum for public debate and action in support of research, patient care, and philanthropy. In short, a must read for anyone involved in treating, supporting, or living with chronic disease." — C. GARRISON FATHMAN, M.D., CHAIRMAN, CENTER FOR CLINICAL IMMUNOLOGY, STANFORD UNIVERSITY SCHOOL OF MEDICINE

"What a wonderful experience, what a wonderful message of hope! I really admire a doctor who, when he couldn't practice medicine due to the disease he suffered, found another way to help patients and bring them hope. I find that truly inspiring, and it encourages me to do the same in my battle against MG. In French we say, 'Help yourself and Heaven will help you!' " — STÉPHANE HUBERTY, M.D., MG PATIENT, CEO, CuraVac, INC., BRUSSELS, BELGIUM

"As the father of a daughter who has myasthenia, I find this book to be a tremendous source of information and encouragement. Hopefully, with the efforts of Dr. Ron Henderson and others, a cure will soon be found." — DENNIS BRAVATA, DENNIS J. BRAVATA APPRAISALS, GRAND RAPIDS, MICHIGAN

"A captivating story of a physician's journey to the other side of the reflex hammer and beyond. Dr. Henderson's observations, lessons, and challenges for change are relevant to all . . . who care for those with chronic diseases." — ROBERT J. FOX, M.D., MULTIPLE SCLEROSIS CLINICIAN AND RESEARCHER, MELLEN CENTER, CLEVELAND CLINIC FOUNDATION, CLEVELAND, OHIO

"Dr. Henderson writes frankly and compassionately about his experiences with MG, describing his first signs of illness, the difficult process of diagnosis, and his search for effective treatment. This book is a must-have companion for anyone with an interest in MG." — LOIS PEDERSEN, M.S., EXECUTIVE DIRECTOR, MYASTHENIA GRAVIS FOUNDATION OF CALIFORNIA

"As an MG patient, I struggle with the day-to-day symptoms, treatment methods, and lack of understanding about MG in both the medical community and the community-at-large. This book is desperately needed." — DONNA NIKOLAS, MG PATIENT, CEO OF GIRL SCOUTS OF MACOMB COUNTY, OTSIKITA COUNCIL, INC., CLINTON TOWNSHIP, MICHIGAN

ATTACKING MYASTHENIA GRAVIS

A Key in the Battle Against Autoimmune Diseases

RONALD E. HENDERSON, M.D.

NEWSOUTH BOOKS
Montgomery

NewSouth Books
105 South Court Street
Montgomery, AL 36104

Library of Congress Cataloguing-in-Publication Data

ISBN 978-1-58838-114-9 (hardcover)
ISBN 978-1-60306-267-1 (paperback)

Design by Randall Williams

Printed in the United States of America

TO

BETH

MY WIFE, MY BEST FRIEND, MY SOUL MATE, AND THE ULTIMATE
CAREGIVER. WITHOUT BETH'S ASSISTANCE, IMPECCABLE CARE,
AND DETAILED ATTENTION, I WOULD NOT BE AS HEALTHY AS I AM
TODAY AND THIS BOOK WOULD NOT HAVE BEEN POSSIBLE.

CONTENTS

INTRODUCTION

This book began as a self-help book in one very specific area. It was designed to help individuals who are battling a chronic muscle-weakness disease called myasthenia gravis (MG), and it was designed to help their families. As the book unfolded, it began taking on "a life of its own." This occurred as I told my own story and also as I interviewed others about their stories. As information accumulated, the book steadily extended well beyond the original scope I initially had in mind.

In its finished version, the book still has as its centerpiece this disease called myasthenia gravis, a rare and little-known neuromuscular, auto-immune disease with which I personally am waging an ongoing battle. However, the centerpiece of myasthenia gravis has taken its place in the midst of lessons that reach far beyond MG.

As I began to recall the story of my own battle against MG, and as three incredible people began sharing with me the stories of their own MG battles, I realized that much of what was pouring forth from all four of us has applications not just to MG but to *all chronic diseases.*

All four of us tell of struggles and triumphs with which I feel many chronic disease patients can identify. All four of us have the same goal that I believe is deeply shared by millions of other chronic disease patients. Our goal is simply this: Although we know we suffer from an ongoing, chronic health problem for which there is treatment but no cure, we have the goal of continuing to live quality, productive lives. We know that to get the most out of life we must put our disease on the back shelf and deal with it only as needed. All four of us know that we have journeyed out of some darkness into light. We know that life for us today is good in spite of our chronic disease. And we know that along the way we have learned lessons we want to share with many others who suffer from a wide range of chronic diseases.

Thus, this book is not just a myasthenia gravis self-help book. It's a chronic disease self-help book.

As this book took on a life of its own, my original missions with the book did not change. At the same time, additional new missions began to take shape.

One of my key original missions was to make the public more aware of myasthenia gravis—to spread an understanding of what MG is, and how it affects those who have it. That mission stays intact. I want anyone who reads this book to learn considerably more about MG. I invite you to learn from a distinguished neurologist who discusses MG diagnosis and treatment, from a brilliant researcher who describes promising MG vaccine research, and from the patients' stories told by my three fellow MG patients and myself.

Another original mission, which also stays intact, was to announce my plans to establish a new foundation that will focus on myasthenia gravis and other autoimmune diseases. I'm very excited about the potential for this foundation and will use this introduction to describe my vision for it.

As for this book's additional missions that relate to the broader picture of chronic diseases, these are a couple that stand out:

One of my additional missions for the book as it relates to the overall chronic disease picture has to do with conveying crucial messages to four key audiences. These four audiences are patients who suffer from chronic diseases, physicians who treat chronic disease patients, caregivers who provide support and care for chronic disease patients, and communities in which these chronic disease patients and their caregivers reside. In formulating and communicating messages to these four audiences, I found myself wearing two hats. One hat is that of a patient waging a battle against a chronic disease. The other hat is that of a physician who practiced medicine for almost three decades and who places heartfelt emphasis on providing each patient with attentive, individualized medical care.

Another of my additional missions for the book as it relates to chronic disease in general has to do with shining the spotlight on what I call "aggravators" and "fixers." Here again, I'm wearing the hats of both patient and physician. When I refer to an aggravator, I'm speaking of something damaging which I personally feel can contribute to making a chronic disease worse and in some cases might even help trigger a disease in the first place. In this book, the spotlight is heavily on one aggravator—stress, or, more specifically, unmanaged stress. When I refer to a fixer, I'm speaking of something positive that can help you fix, or improve, various aspects of your life as a chronic disease patient. This doesn't mean something magical that can fix your chronic disease to the extent of curing it. Instead, it relates to helpmates that can improve your ability to live with your chronic disease and make your life more enjoyable despite your chronic disease. This book focuses in on two fixers. One fixer is exercise. The other fixer is maintaining a positive attitude.

Increasing Awareness about Myasthenia Gravis

A deep need exists in this nation to increase awareness about the disease known as myasthenia gravis, or MG—a disease with a name that means "grave muscle weakness." This need for MG awareness exists not only in the general public but in the medical community as well.

Many patients suffering from MG endure months or even years of symptoms without obtaining a diagnosis, including some who go from doctor to doctor complaining of symptoms. One needs only to read the story of Kelley Haughey in this book to get a taste of what some MG patients have endured in the past (and still endure) in trying to find a medical explanation for their strange sets of muscle-weakness symptoms.

I am sympathetic to the challenges faced by today's medical schools in trying to compress increasing amounts of knowledge into the four-year curriculum for physicians' basic medical education. Being aware of this challenge, I realize that rare diseases such as MG can claim little time and attention in the broad spectrum of medical schools' curricula. Also, I am sympathetic to the fact that one of the early symptoms of MG often is simply acute fatigue, a feeling of being very tired. Since that's a symptom which can be associated with a wide range of health problems, a physician has to have his antennae up for MG in order to even consider that diagnosis as an option to investigate. These are among the reasons a great deal of this book is devoted to MG awareness. I want the book to serve as one tool to help fill a gap. The goal is that many medical students, residents, and practicing physicians will become more aware of myasthenia gravis through reading this book.

Too, it is my intention that, through this book, many MG patients and their families will become more familiar with this disease. The book can be used by MG patients as a guide to help them take better control of their own disease.

Communicating to All Chronic Disease Patients

Although all the patients' stories in this book come from those who are suffering from myasthenia gravis, these MG patients raise issues, concerns, and needs that no doubt will ring a bell with patients suffering from many other chronic health problems.

If you have a chronic health problem, you might well find food for thought in the pages of this book. When I use the designation of "a patient suffering from a chronic health problem," I'm referring to someone who is dealing with a health condition for which, at this time, he or she can't go out and take a magical pill or other treatment and make it go away. Even though the individual can look forward to better treatments, and in some cases even anticipate the possibility of a cure, at the present time the challenge is to build a quality life in spite of the chronic health problem.

You might be waging a long-term battle with diabetes, rheumatoid arthritis, multiple sclerosis, lupus, or a wide range of other autoimmune diseases for which there are only treatments and no cures.

You could be fighting a chronic battle with one of the many types of cancer.

Or you could be trying to carve out a new life for yourself after sustaining disability resulting from an accident, stroke, heart disease, or a devastating illness.

Regardless of the nature of your chronic health problem, you share some common bonds with others who have other types of chronic health problems. These are some of the issues, concerns, and needs raised in this book by MG patients—issues, concerns, and needs that I feel have universal chronic disease application:

The patients in this book talk about the value of quality, personalized healthcare to diagnose and treat them. They talk of the value of health professionals who really listen to them, who treat them as individuals.

They talk about the value of family and friends to understand them, listen to them, and stand by them. They talk of the need for quality caregivers.

They talk of the need to educate themselves about their disease, to empower themselves with knowledge.

And they talk about very personal emotional and spiritual issues. They talk about times during their chronic disease battles when they have been hurt, depressed, and/or frustrated; and they relate how they have dealt with those valleys. They talk about how they have emerged with a positive attitude as their friend. They talk about spirituality and what that means to them.

In recalling their own personal stories, the patients in this book indeed address key issues that bind all patients with chronic health problems.

Establishing a New Foundation

This book is a key tool in introducing the International Autoimmune Disease Research Foundation, a new not-for-profit foundation devoted to myasthenia gravis and related autoimmune diseases.

I recently set up this foundation because I am driven to find a cure for MG and hopeful of unlocking doors that lead to breakthroughs with related autoimmune diseases. The foundation will serve as a catalyst and vehicle for research in the autoimmune disease arena.

By "autoimmune disease" I refer to any of a wide range of diseases in which the body's immune system in some way turns against an individual. When this happens, a disease process is born out of abnormal circumstances in the human body that are the opposite of the natural way the immune system is supposed to function. Ideally, your immune system is supposed to protect you. But when it turns against you, the result can be a disease such as myasthenia gravis, multiple sclerosis, type I diabetes, Guillain-Barré syndrome, lupus, rheumatoid arthritis, or any one of a number of others. As for what goes wrong to make the immune system turn against an individual, there are many research theories that can vary from disease to disease. Among the theories are damage resulting from bacterial or viral infections, stress, exposure to toxins, genetic predisposition, and just plain unknown causes.

The foundation will have myasthenia gravis, or MG, as its first research priority. I want the foundation to focus first on MG not because I have this disease, but because many scientists view MG as being arguably the best understood of all autoimmune diseases at the pathophysiological level. Since MG is well understood in comparison to many of its sister autoimmune diseases, I am convinced that MG can serve as somewhat of an autoimmune research model. It is a significant part of my vision that some of the MG research projects funded by the new foundation will uncover knowledge not only about MG but about other autoimmune diseases as well. For example, I think one of the first projects that should be considered for funding is a myasthenia gravis vaccine basic research project headed by Dr. J. Edwin Blalock at the University of Alabama at Birmingham (UAB), a project described in detail in this book. Typical of the potential "spillover" effect of MG research into other autoimmune disease areas, Dr. Blalock is expressing optimism that his vaccine research could have future application to other autoimmune diseases in addition to MG.

Although this foundation will focus heavily on both basic and clinical scientific research, the foundation's missions will not be limited to these traditional research areas. For instance, the foundation could sponsor research in the area of epidemiology—looking at the incidence and distribution of autoimmune diseases such as MG.

In addition to focusing on research, I also envision this foundation undertaking projects to directly assist patients with their treatments. Along this line, one of the areas I'm interested in exploring is for the foundation to assume the role of "facilitator" in helping medically needy MG patients gain access to the medications they need. In the treatment of myasthenia gravis some of the medications are quite expensive. I envision this new foundation taking on the role of connector between patients and pharmaceutical companies, to help develop programs that make available discounted or free medications for patients in need.

Over the past several months, I have spent considerable time developing and refining my vision for this foundation in which I so strongly believe. I began formulating the vision as soon as my doctors and I began to be successful in getting my own MG condition under control. It was as though I felt driven to take the lead in setting up such a foundation. It somehow seemed that it would be a shame for me not to use my background to try to do some good in the area of chronic autoimmune diseases. After all, it was a chronic autoimmune disease, namely MG, that forced me to retire from the practice of medicine in the prime of my career. I can identify with the havoc a chronic disease can create in someone's life. I've decided it's time for me to go back to work, in a different role—this time as founder and leader of this new foundation.

I believe my background has prepared me for a leadership role in the foundation. Throughout my medical and entrepreneurial career, I've tried to improve systems and quality. To accomplish that through design of systems and programs, I've worked in founding or cofounding (and in some cases managing) entities such as a women's healthcare center, a professional liability insurance company, a health maintenance organization, a prototype outpatient surgery center, and a physician practice management company. I've pursued concurrent goals that include improving convenience in healthcare, enhancing quality of care for patients, and at the same time keeping costs in line. Now that I am suffering from a chronic disease and understand it both from a patient's view and a physician's view, I think it's natural for me to look at trying to improve the system that supports chronic disease patients.

In launching any new major initiative, it is always crucial to recruit topflight individuals as part of the team. I plan to do that with the foundation. In addition to having an experienced operating board, the foundation will have a respected lay advisory board and a high-profile scientific advisory board.

Serving on the lay advisory board will be business and civic leaders with distinctive track records. They will be called upon for their guidance from the points of view of such relevant entities and groups as patients, family members and other caregivers of patients, social service agencies, healthcare providers, communities at large, business and industry, and philanthropy.

As for the scientific advisory board, this will be a board made up of extremely knowledgeable clinicians and bench scientists. Members of this board will be well versed in the diseases the foundation addresses, they will be impartial, and they will be credible. It will be their mission to guide the foundation in wisely allocating the funds we raise for research.

Reaching Out to Target Audiences

Through this book, crucial messages are directed to several audiences. In a section of the book entitled "Messages for Key Audiences," I elaborate on issues as they apply to each of four audiences in particular. Those audiences are chronic disease patients, physicians, caregivers, and communities.

I believe strongly in these messages and want to pinpoint central themes within the messages for each of the four audiences:

For the patient suffering from a chronic disease, it is my intention that as you read the book you will feel more informed and more motivated. Personally, I feel that the words on these pages can help empower you to take charge, to take more control of managing your disease. If you already are exerting some control in your own disease management, perhaps this book can motivate you to take even more steps to learn about your disease, to seek out solutions to minimize your symptoms, and to maximize your positive attitude. In this book's chapter on diagnosing and treating MG, neurologist Dr. Shin Oh provides helpful information. Also, the MG patients who share their stories offer valuable insights. Here again, the material dealing directly with MG offers many lessons that can be used not just by MG patients, but by all patients who are dealing with chronic health problems. For example, Baptist minister Dr. Steve Gaines, an MG patient, provides great insight on the subject of re-evaluating and sometimes rearranging one's priorities in life. Dr. Gaines tells his own story of how dealing with a chronic disease has motivated him to prioritize in order to use his diminished supply of energy in the wisest, most efficient manner. That's something that applies to many chronic disease patients, not just to MG patients!

For physicians who treat chronic disease patients, it is hoped this book will motivate you to try to fill some of what I view as "holes" in our healthcare system in terms of chronic disease management. There are a lot of isolated chronic disease patients out there today who are falling through the cracks of a healthcare system that is fraught with problems and broken parts. You as an individual physician do not have to be part of the problem. You can be part of the solution. I issue this challenge to each and every physician who is providing medical care to chronic disease patients: Individualize the medical care you provide to each chronic disease patient. Don't treat the patient with a pat template. For each patient, physicians should individualize and personalize the medical care, and then micromanage the rendering of that care.

For caregivers of chronically ill people, I hope this book will impress upon you how essential you are, and how effective you can be. If caregiving is performed correctly, with knowledge, love, and respect, it can be extremely helpful to the patient and very fulfilling for the caregiver. Over the years in my role as a physician, I have been favorably impressed time and again, hundreds of times, in seeing what a tremendous amount of knowledge and insight caregivers can absorb in such a short period of time! Because of the fragmented way much of the healthcare system is set up today, it's vital that a chronic disease patient's care be managed with active participation by the patient himself or his primary caregiver. The ideal way, whenever possible, is to have active participation by *both* the patient and his primary caregiver.

And, finally, for communities, I hope this book provides inspiration for citizens to come together to offer programs to help chronically ill patients and their families. There is not a community in America that does not have this need. And every community in America, no matter how big or how small, no matter how wealthy or how modest, can come together in some way to help meet that need. Never underestimate the power of one individual.

Casting a Spotlight on Stress

As you read this book's personal stories that are related by MG patients, you will see the subject of stress crop up time and again. For example, you will see situations in which myasthenia gravis first appeared in individuals' lives soon after these individuals had sustained grave physical, emotional, or mental stresses. Coincidence? Perhaps. Perhaps not. You also will see situations in which it has been crucial for an individual to bring stress under control in his or her life in order to manage the MG.

Speaking as both a physician and a chronic disease patient, I urge you to commit yourself to using parts of this book as a lesson in stress management.

I think it behooves all of us to think about stress in our lives and how we can best manage it. We all have stress. Learning how to manage stress effectively is the challenge. In some cases, taking specific steps in our lives to decrease stress, to prevent or minimize it, becomes the task at hand.

It is my strong opinion that in relation to all autoimmune diseases, stress probably plays a big part in injuring the immune system. This is an area of sufficient interest to draw the attention of many researchers. I believe that stress is a contributing factor, an aggravator, in the onset of some chronic diseases—diseases of autoimmune nature, and also some others as well. And I know I will encounter little argument that stress management certainly is important in properly managing those diseases once they have been diagnosed.

The longer we live, the more concerns we have, the more complicated society becomes, stress becomes an increasingly negative influence on our health. Many factors contribute: The fast pace at which we live. The breakdown of our family units. The decline of togetherness in our communities. Escalating societal problems, including spousal and child abuse and addictions to alcohol, illegal drugs, and/or prescription medications.

Then there's the added reality that we are an aging society. Many of us are living longer than did our ancestors. The longer you live, the higher are your chances that you will encounter additional major stresses. Also, the longer you live, the higher are your chances that you will be diagnosed with a chronic disease. Often the challenges of managing the two—stress and chronic disease—go hand in hand.

Getting in a Plug for Exercise

Anyone who has ever known me would not believe his or her eyes if I wrote a book that did not include a pitch for regular, disciplined exercise. My lifelong belief in and practice of regular physical exercise is widely known to my family, friends, professional colleagues, and also to my many patients over the years.

Eight years ago, when I began experiencing severe symptoms of what proved to be myasthenia gravis, I was forced for a time to give up my daily hour-long exercise regimen. It was a big loss to me. There's no doubt in my mind that it affected me adversely in terms of physical stamina, mental quickness, and emotional well-being. However, for a time I was in a "catch-22 situation." On the one hand, I needed the exercise more than ever to build back my strength and physical stamina that had been depleted by MG. However, on the other hand, one of the key symptoms of myasthenia gravis in its acute stage is that often you are robbed of the physical stamina and strength you must have to do the exercise in the first place. That's where I was for a while. (That catch-22 situation might well ring a familiar bell with some of you who are dealing with acute stages of a chronic health problem.)

As a part of traveling my own road from having been very sick with MG to currently having my disease under control, I am now back to a regular daily exercise program. Today I subscribe even more avidly than ever to the benefits that exercise brings. I'm convinced my exercise program is one of the "fixers" that's helping me to live an active life in spite of the MG.

If you are a chronic disease patient reading this book, I hope you are motivated to investigate exercise as a part of your daily regimen. Of course, you must consult with your physician before undertaking any exercise program. And situations will vary greatly from patient to patient in terms of your capacity for exercise and what type of exercise program you should pursue.

In regard to exercise for the chronic disease patient, I have a few thoughts for you:

- Even if your chronic disease in its most acute stages deprives you of your ability to exercise for a period of time, that doesn't mean that things have to remain that way. As you get a handle on your disease, revisit the option of exercise.

• Exercising means different things to different people. Even if you have a health condition that means you cannot exercise your entire body, investigate the option of exercising parts of your body.

• Seek expert professional advice about your exercise program.

I'm not the only one in this book who is high on exercise. When you read the story of family physician Dr. Steve TePastte and his own battle against myasthenia gravis, you'll see what I mean!

Just in terms of myasthenia gravis patients alone, I have seen cases in which patients reported significant improvement in the way they felt just through initiating a carefully controlled daily regimen of exercise, balanced with periods of rest.

There's nothing like finishing an exercise session and having that in-control, "I-am-pleasantly-tired" feeling. Exercise is good for your body physically. It strengthens your body. It gives you energy. It's a tool in keeping your weight under control. I'm among those who are convinced that exercise is a friend to your immune system and helps you to fight off health problems. Also, there's no doubt that exercise stimulates you mentally and soothes you emotionally. Exercise is exhilarating. It helps you to feel better. It helps you to have a more positive view of yourself and a more positive view of life in general.

Facing Life's Problems with a Positive Attitude

I believe in it. Kelley Haughey believes in it. Dr. Steve TePastte be-lieves in it. And Dr. Steve Gaines believes in it. All four of us who tell our stories about confronting myasthenia gravis are in agreement that it's the way to go.

If you're not already trying it, all of us recommend it. If you are, don't stop.

"It" has to do with facing life, including its problems, with a positive attitude.

As Kelley, the two Steves, and I relate our stories of confronting myasthenia gravis, the theme of positive thinking is a recurrent one.

That doesn't mean we haven't had our "down days." Oh yes, the down days have been there with all of us. But, in order to see our way through to brighter days, a positive spirit ultimately has had to prevail. And, for each of us, a positive spirit *has* prevailed.

I've said it thousands of times. This book says it in many ways: *It's not so much what happens in your life that matters; it's how you view what happens in your life and how you deal with it that really matters.*

Above all, as you read this book I hope you become convinced, or reconvinced, of the necessity of approaching your life and its challenges with a positive attitude. No matter what challenges you might face, life looks better and works better if you view the glass as being not half-empty, but instead as being half-full. I hope in these pages you will see many ways that you can use your persistence and tenacity to turn your own life's lemons into lemonade.

Ronald E. Henderson, M.D.

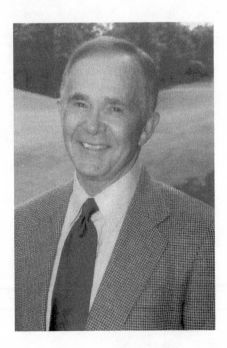

ACKNOWLEDGMENTS

I gladly take this opportunity to express gratitude to several individuals who have contributed in a variety of ways to this book about a chronic neuromuscular, autoimmune disease known as myasthenia gravis, or MG.

As you, the reader, make your journey through the reading of the book, you will see how five individuals have joined with me in supplying core content. To each of them, I express my heartfelt appreciation. From a content perspective, the book has been written as one of both personal inspiration and specific lifestyle and disease management information. In the process, I have interviewed individuals who have offered diverse insights. My thanks go first to three fellow MG patients who, like myself, share the personal stories of how they have battled, and continue to battle, this disease. These three MG patients are Kelley Haughey, Dr. Steve TePastte, and Dr. Steve Gaines. Next, to neurologist Dr. Shin Oh, I express gratitude for his insights into the diagnosing and treating of MG. Finally, to researcher/immunologist Dr. Ed Blalock, I say thank-you for an explanation of his MG vaccine research project which this book spotlights.

We all are aware that while part of the making of a book is centered in content, another important part is embedded in book-packaging features that determine how a book's cover and pages are designed and visually presented to the human eye. I feel the production of this book has benefited greatly from the consultation, advice, and design services of Randall Williams and Suzanne La Rosa, associated with NewSouth, Inc., and its NewSouth Books imprint in Montgomery, Alabama.

I express my gratitude to the book's proofreaders, Lynn Edge and Maria Coyle.

And my thanks go to Anita Smith for her invaluable editorial and organizational help with this book.

FOREWORD

PHILIP D. WALTON, M.D.

I first met Dr. Ron Henderson in the spring of 1969, when I was a third-year student at the University of Alabama School of Medicine in Birmingham, Alabama. The first day I saw Dr. Henderson, he was consulting on a case at University Hospital involving a patient who had a complex medical problem. He came from his office at St. Vincent's Hospital to review the case with several of us who were medical students and residents. I never will forget how impressed I was with him, mainly because of his brilliant and quick mind. It was obvious that he was a well-trained, compassionate and caring physician. He clearly exhibited good judgment in taking care of patients. It was on this day at University Hospital when I first began seriously considering obstetrics and gynecology (OB-GYN) as my future specialty. After that I referred to Dr. Henderson a new patient—my wife, Jane.

While I was a medical student, as part of my training I rotated through St. Vincent's Hospital, Dr. Henderson's primary hospital of practice. For my residency, I did select OB-GYN as my specialty. During this time I had the opportunity to interact with Dr. Henderson and his partner, Dr. Ernest Moore.

Needless to say, I was extremely pleased and honored when Dr. Henderson called me in early 1975 to ask if I would be interested in joining him and Dr. Moore in practice. At the time he called me, he was a patient in St. Vincent's Hospital, recuperating from serious injuries he had sustained in an automobile accident in December 1974.

As soon as I completed two years of active duty with the United States Air Force, in June 1976, I joined Dr. Henderson and Dr. Moore in practice. That marked the beginning of an 18-year professional relationship I had with Ron Henderson as his medical partner; it marked the beginning of a close friendship that continues today.

Since I know Ron Henderson well—as a physician and as a person—in these few pages I want to introduce you, the reader of this book, to the Ron Henderson I know.

I want you to meet Ron Henderson, the visionary.

One of the great attributes of Dr. Ron Henderson is the impact he has had as a visionary. He not only has the ability to cast the vision; he also has the ability to implement the vision. I saw that firsthand as I watched Ron function as chief executive officer of Henderson & Walton Women's Center in Birmingham. As we built a practice that was both exemplary and large (currently 18 physicians), Ron charted our course with his phenomenal ability to think outside the lines. Under his leadership, we built a practice based on the "Four C's of Healthcare"—compassionate, competent, cost-effective, and convenient. We built the practice around a mission statement with the Golden Rule as a cornerstone: "Do unto others as you would have them do unto you." We built it around the philosophy of treating the patient first as your friend. In keeping with our goal to provide comprehensive care and to make medical care convenient for the patient, Ron coined the phrase "one-stop shopping." He felt we should go beyond offering the conventional OB-GYN screening services such as mammograms and Pap smears. Under his leadership, we added services such as cholesterol screening and nutritional and psychological counseling. We even began offering sigmoidoscopies, virtually unheard of in an OB-GYN practice. (Within a few days of instituting this we diagnosed an early colon cancer.) Prior to becoming a specialist in obstetrics and gynecology, Ron had been a family doctor in a small Alabama town for two years. He understood the value of comprehensive care. Ron said we should focus not just on a patient's OB-GYN needs, but instead look at the entire patient in relation to her overall physical, mental, and emotional well-being. In addition, Ron led our practice in reaching out to communities within a 60-mile radius of Birmingham that did not have sufficient OB-GYN services. The result was the birth of a network. We set up Henderson & Walton Women's Center satellite offices and now have satellites in seven Alabama towns.

I want those of you reading this book to meet Ron Henderson, the leader in organized medicine.

When I first joined Ron in practice, he already had been serving for several years as a member of the powerful State Committee of Public Health, which in Alabama functions as the State Board of Health and governs the state's public health system. Also during that period, Ron was on the forefront of leadership in the health planning movement as a member of the State Health Planning and Development Agency Board.

Then, in the early 1980s, when he became president of the Medical Association of the State of Alabama (MASA), Ron had arrived at a position in organized medicine in which he could exert tremendous influence statewide during extraordinarily changing times in the practice of medicine. Ron had accurate perceptions of where the practice of medicine was headed; I've said often that Ron was several years ahead of his time with his insights. During the year he led the state's medical association, Ron shared his insights with Alabama physicians through his speeches and widely read articles he wrote for MASA's journal. He shared insights that physicians were glad to hear, and he also shared insights that some did not want to hear. For example, the title of one of the articles Ron wrote during that period was "Smile More, Earn Less." Ron knew that reimbursement for physicians' services was on the way down, that physicians' incomes were about to drop. He was urging physicians to prepare to face that unpleasant reality while displaying a positive attitude to patients and professional colleagues.

Ron was so progressive that there were those who felt he was a natural to become president of the American Medical Association (AMA). In the mid to late 1980s, he seemed well on his way. He became a member of AMA's House of Delegates, vice chairman of AMA's Council on Medical Service, and chairman of that council's Subcommittee on Financing Healthcare for the Elderly. Ron was holding prestigious positions that gave him a national platform. Yet he felt torn between his desire to continue moving up the AMA ladder and spending more time at home with his two great loves—his family and his practice. He also was confronting the reality of the bureaucracy that was involved in the AMA. Ron came to the decision that the structure was too complex to absorb the changes he felt were needed. He decided to pull back from his AMA activities in order to focus his full attention on his medical practice and innovative healthcare programs he had been launching in Alabama.

I want you to meet Ron Henderson, the agent of change who became founder and cofounder of programs to improve the healthcare system.

In 1976, Ron became one of the cofounders of Mutual Assurance Society of Alabama, a physician-owned-and-operated liability insurance company. Once again, because of Ron's perception of where medical care was heading, he was among a few physicians able to see what was on the horizon in terms of the malpractice crisis. As a cofounder of Mutual Assurance, Ron was one of those who envisioned and implemented this liability company for doctors in Alabama. This was a company that would be operated in an efficient, cost-effective manner and would serve as a defense strategy against malpractice cases. A successful and model plan from its inception, Mutual Assurance has expanded its scope to include other areas of coverage and has broadened its geographical base far beyond the state of Alabama.

In 1983, Ron became one of the cofounders of the Birmingham Surgical Center, the first freestanding outpatient surgical care facility in the Southeast. The facility was founded early in the beginning of a national trend for some surgical cases to be performed in an outpatient setting. This concept called for patients to be able to undergo certain surgical procedures with a few hours' stay in an outpatient facility, without having to be admitted to the hospital. The concept was directed toward surgical cases that were not complex and which in many cases were elective. Advantages to the patients were savings of both time and money. At a time when many hospitals were resisting this movement, Ron was among a small group of physicians in Birmingham who believed in the concept enough to invest time and resources to make it happen. This center became a model, and it continues to operate today as one of the most successful outpatient care centers of its type in the Southeast.

In 1984, Ron made more history when he became the founder and chief executive officer of Southeast Health Plan, the first physician-owned combination independent practice association and health maintenance organization in the Southeast. Ron believed strongly there should be an alternative, a new approach, to the way health insurance was structured. He felt there was major room for improvement in terms of premium cost, reimbursement to hospitals and physicians, and emphasis on preventive medicine. He knew there had to be a more efficient way to manage those dollars than currently was being done. In the several years that Southeast Health Plan operated, it set major positive examples—including linking lower premiums to subscribers' healthy lifestyles. Ron's goal was that this approach would place such strong emphasis on preventive care that it would keep patients healthier. There is no doubt Southeast Health Plan made an impact in focusing more conventional health-insurance attention on patients' healthy lifestyles, such as not smoking and being conscious of proper diet and exercise.

Then, in 1992, Ron founded MediSphere Corporation, Inc., a physician practice management (PPM) company that ultimately represented a number of physician groups in Alabama, Georgia, Mississippi, and North Carolina. Ron clearly saw there were more efficient ways to manage and grow physician practices—if they could consolidate some of their operations and address business goals such as economies of scale. MediSphere later merged with a Nashville, Tennessee-based PPM company to become MediSphere Health Partners. When Ron founded MediSphere, he again was several years ahead of his time and structured what was a new paradigm shift in the way physicians practiced medicine.

I want you to meet Ron Henderson, an example of boundless energy, dedicated work ethic, consistent self-discipline, and positive attitude.

During the years that Ron was leading us in the building of Henderson & Walton Women's Center and was involved in so many outside activities, he had what seemed to be unlimited energy. In fact, I've never known anyone who had as much stamina as he did.

Added to his natural energy level was his ability to function well with only five to six hours of sleep at night. Add to this his positive attitude toward work; he loved his work, he worked hard and steadily, and he knew how to manage his time. Too, he approached every day with an incredible amount of self-discipline, not only with his work but also in managing his health and fitness—such as eating a healthy diet, exercising, and keeping his weight down.

Ron would arise in the mornings around 4 o'clock. Before coming to work, he engaged in an intensive hour-long exercise program. He usually was the first physician in the practice to arrive at work in the morning and was the last to leave in the evening. Also, he typically saw more patients than anyone else in the practice, even while handling his many administrative and outside commitments.

He was so healthy that most of the time he felt great. On rare occasions when he didn't feel his best, he just kept going. He had a mental outlook so positive that he could overlook minor aches and pains, and that continues today. Ron felt there must be extenuating circumstances for not going to work. He set the standard, and the rest of us in the practice followed that standard. Be it snow or be it ice, we went to work. The patients might not be there, but we were there—because Ron was there. Ron also set the standard about when to leave at the end of the day. You left not according to the time as told by the clock; you left after all the patients' needs had been addressed.

Even though Ron practiced extraordinary self-discipline in his daily life, he still had it in him to go even further when he felt the need. When he was involved in an accident in 1974, he suffered injuries that required extensive rehabilitation—including a crushed pelvis, a fractured left femur, and 10 broken ribs. He went the extra mile with his own workout regimen long after his initial recovery. Part of his routine was to swim early each morning at home in a pool he had installed specifically to help with his rehabilitation. I recall Ron's unwavering dedication to his swimming regimen, even on the coldest of winter mornings. Although the pool was heated and covered, he faced the reality of a cold walk to the house once he got out of the pool.

I want you to meet Dr. Ron Henderson, a compassionate physician and a skilled surgeon.

Ron was a master surgeon, known for his skill and speed in the operating room. I now see patients that Ron operated on years ago who still are enjoying excellent results from his surgery. As a great teacher in the operating room, he emphasized several important surgical principles. Among them were that a surgeon should never have any wasted motion in the operating room, everything the surgeon does must have a purpose, and the goal is to operate on the patient skillfully while using as little operative time as possible. He knew that when you prevented wasted motion, the patient lost less blood, suffered less trauma to the tissues, and recovered more quickly.

Ron was a physician who was much-loved and much-respected by his patients. He has been retired now for almost eight years, and still we have many patients who ask about Dr. Henderson. Ron rendered excellent care to his patients. He just loved the practice of medicine so much and cared so deeply for his patients that they could *feel* his caring. Ron had a gift, an absolute gift, for focusing on a patient and giving that individual his undivided attention during her visit with him. With all the responsibilities that Ron faced—running our practice, and being involved in so many outside activities—there were tremendous demands on his time with meetings, phone calls, etc. That meant that sometimes Ron's patients had to wait to see him. But after a patient finished an appointment, she was likely to forget or not mind that she had waited, because he had given such undivided attention to her health needs.

I want you to meet Ron Henderson, the "people person."

In my opinion, one of the reasons Ron always has been such a leader is that he loves people, is energized by them, and is able to motivate them to do their best. Since he is such a people person, Ron believes that the talents of each individual should be recognized and appreciated. In our practice at Henderson & Walton Women's Center, we adopted Ron's philosophy that we did not refer to staff members who worked there as "employees" but instead as "associates." He made it a point to communicate frequently with associates about the direction of the practice. Ron likes to see people grow personally and professionally. For example, in our practice Ron led the way for many of our physicians and associates to take the Dale Carnegie course and also to learn the theories of motivational speaker Zig Ziglar.

I want you to meet Ron Henderson, the humanitarian.

Ron is modest and low-key about the many contributions he makes to the betterment of society and to helping individuals. He spearheaded the fund drive to raise the monies to endow a chair in anesthesiology at the University of Alabama School of Medicine, a part of the University of Alabama at Birmingham (UAB). That chair was named in honor of our beloved friend and colleague, pioneer anesthesiologist Alfred "Freddy" Habeeb. Ron has contributed both time and money as a board member of the St. Vincent's Hospital Foundation, including aiding tremendously in the project to build a lodge for patients and their families. Too, there have been times when I have known him to loan or give money confidentially to people in need.

I want you to meet Ron Henderson, my longtime partner and close friend.

There is nothing I wouldn't do for Ron Henderson, and I know there is nothing he wouldn't do for me. We have a friendship so close it's more like we are brothers. Over the years, we have laughed together, we have cried together, we have worked hard together, and we have spent long hours together. We have shared fun times together, we've been on the water and in the airplane and ridden horses together, our families have spent time together, our children became good friends and his children even babysat for mine. Jane and I have four children, and Ron delivered three of the four; he would have delivered all four except one was born the year Jane and I were in North Carolina for my internship. Ron and I have been there for each other when there were happy times to share, we have been there for each other when we lost parents, and we have been there for each other in times of need. After I fell and broke my elbow in 1977, I arrived at the hospital to find Ron waiting for me—not inside the emergency room, but out in the hospital parking lot even before I reached the emergency room!

As partners in our rapidly growing medical practice, I always called Ron "Partner" and he called me "Chief." In our practice, we cared for a large volume of patients, and we cared for many high-risk patients referred to us with complex medical problems. We turned to each other for consultation. We asked each another questions such as: "This is what I'm thinking; do you agree with that?" And we enjoyed being partners and assisting each other in the operating room. We were compatible; our movements and our surgical approaches matched. When Ron retired from the practice of medicine in late 1994, it was emotional for both of us. I shall never forget the last day we did a surgical case together. We had known that day was approaching, that the hour was coming. So it arrived. He had a 7 a.m. case, and I was assisting. We both were painfully aware that would be his last surgical case before retiring. But we didn't mention it when we arrived in the hospital surgical area and saw each other that morning. We just walked in like we'd normally done thousands of times before. We got into our scrub suits, shoes, hats, and masks. We scrubbed together, talked about the things we normally would talk about, and went in and did the case. Then, after completing our last case together, we went to my office. There I presented him with a gift made just for him. I had found a pair of Mayo surgical scissors with gold-plated handles. I had the scissors mounted on a wooden stand, with a plaque inscribed with this message: "To my Partner—the best." That was a time we will always remember. When Ron Henderson left the practice of medicine, it was the end of an era.

I want to introduce you to Ron Henderson, the author of this book.

Since Ron seldom complained about anything, I knew he was both concerned and puzzled when he confided to me in 1994 that he was feeling an unexplained loss of energy. For the first time ever, his exercise regimen was leaving him exhausted. And, as time went on, he began feeling a peculiar weakness in his neck muscles and was having trouble holding his head erect. Still, Ron maintained that positive personality, kept that smile on his face, and said upbeat things like "We're going to get this done!" and "Oh, I'll get a good night's sleep tonight and I'll be fine tomorrow."

Today we know that the reason for this unusual muscle weakness and fatigue lay in the fact that Ron had, and still has, the chronic neuromuscular disease known as myasthenia gravis, or MG. Although he did not know at the time that he had myasthenia gravis, there's no doubt that the disease's sapping of his strength and energy was the key contributor to his decision in late 1994 to retire from medical practice.

The Ron Henderson I know is still out there doing what he has always professed—that is, turning a negative into a positive. By authoring this book, Ron is converting the unfortunate diagnosis of MG into something good to help many other people. Through this book, he is sharing with others the tremendous knowledge he has gained since being diagnosed with MG.

Once his diagnosis was confirmed, Ron could have taken the attitude of focusing mostly on himself. But that's not the Ron Henderson I've known all these years. He focused on himself only long enough to work with his physicians to get his disease under control, which thankfully has occurred. And then, feeling a renewal of that old energy, in typical fashion he began focusing on others. That shows in this book.

Since Ron's brilliant mind is never still, once he was diagnosed he began learning all he could about MG. Today I think Ron Henderson's knowledge of systemic myasthenia gravis probably rivals that of many neurologists and other experts across the country. Too, I think Ron has learned and grown on the emotional and spiritual side. As strong as he was prior to MG—and he indeed was strong—I think he's even stronger today. I believe having this disease has given him new perspectives on life that he probably never would have had otherwise. In this book Ron is converting his knowledge and his experiences into ways to inform and help others.

I strongly feel this book will do a great deal to raise awareness about myasthenia gravis by helping people to be more easily diagnosed, by heightening awareness among physicians, and by inspiring and informing patients and their caregivers as well. Also, I think it will help by generating interest in support of research aimed at finding new treatments, and perhaps even a cure, for MG.

Myasthenia gravis has many challenges in common with other autoimmune diseases, as well as other chronic diseases of many types. In this book, I think there are lessons of value for millions who live daily with chronic health problems.

All in all, I predict that through this book Dr. Ronald Earl Henderson, who already has touched so many, is destined to touch even more lives than we could possibly imagine.

Dr. Philip D. Walton is the senior physician at Henderson & Walton Women's Center in Birmingham, Alabama. He is a former medical partner and a longtime friend and colleague of this book's author.

ATTACKING MYASTHENIA GRAVIS

PART ONE

DR. RON HENDERSON
AND MYASTHENIA GRAVIS

I

SEARCHING FOR A DIAGNOSIS

All my life I had heard people comment on my high energy level.

"Ron, you're an incredibly high-energy guy!"

"How do you maintain that schedule of yours? I just don't see how you do it!"

"Don't you ever take a breather?"

Who knows what accounted for all that energy? Likely part of it was genes, part living a healthy lifestyle, part the way I was reared. My dad was a farmer with a strong, disciplined work ethic. I grew up on the farm, where I learned to start working before daybreak and not to let up. My body required only five to six hours of sleep per night, and that helped productivity.

Too, due to the way I was wired, work and energy fed one another. I had the energy to do a lot of work, and then work itself was energizing to me. So the more I worked, the more I would work. Energy fed work, work produced energy, and that energy fed more work. I liked having a lot of balls in the air at once, liked wearing many hats—hats involving both medicine and entrepreneurial ventures.

In February 1994, when the first symptoms hit me of what 21 long months later would be diagnosed as myasthenia gravis, the balls I had in the air were many.

I was a practicing physician (obstetrician-gynecologist, or OB-GYN) and chief executive officer of Henderson & Walton Women's Center in Birmingham, Alabama. That OB-GYN practice had its roots in the 1970s practice that I had founded solo and to which I initially added Dr. Ernie Moore and then Dr. Phil Walton. By 1994, the practice had grown into

a 15-physician organization, with Birmingham headquarters and satellite offices in six Alabama towns, plus extensive on-site ancillary services
that molded it into a unique "one-stop shopping" women's healthcare
center. Totally physician-owned with no co-ownership by a hospital
or health system, this center had become the largest independent OB-
GYN practice of its type in the nation. For me to sit at the helm of this
center's administration required that a steady percentage of my time be
devoted to my role as CEO. In my role as a practicing physician, I had
ceased doing obstetrics several years before; but my patient-care schedule
always was overbooked with gynecology patients. Included among my
patients were large numbers of referrals—often patients with complex
problems, including some who had suffered complications from prior
surgery elsewhere and had been referred to me for corrective surgery.

My big entrepreneurial interest at the time was MediSphere Corporation, Inc., a physician practice management (PPM) company I had
founded a couple of years before. We had gotten in early on the PPM
movement and MediSphere Corporation was showing much promise. We
had what I felt was a unique, high-value model that offered innovative
development and administrative plans to manage and expand practices
for primary-care doctors. The model allowed the physicians complete
autonomy in medical decisions. Since Henderson & Walton Women's
Center had been such a successful high-profile model from both a patient
care and business view, we had many primary-care doctors interested in
exploring an association with MediSphere; this included OB/GYNs,
internists, and pediatricians. To divide my time efficiently between my
practice and MediSphere, I had located the MediSphere offices three
floors above the offices of Henderson & Walton Women's Center. As
another timesaver, I had become an instrument-rated pilot and was able
to pilot my plane to transport me and other MediSphere staff members
on quick out-of-town business trips.

Then there was the farm. For a number of years my wife, Beth, and
I had gradually expanded our Twin Valley Farms. That's our farm property near Prattville, Alabama, some 80 miles south of Birmingham; it's
located a few miles from the farm where I grew up and a few miles from

the home where Beth grew up. As we had expanded that property, Twin Valley had crossed the line from being just a pleasure place to becoming a thriving farm business. Our farm product was different from that of my dad's day; he produced crops, we produced beef. Since the farm had become such an active business by the 1990s, and also since my mother and Beth's mother both were widowed and still lived in Prattville, Beth and I spent as much weekend time there as we could. In fact, we had elected not to maintain a vacation home at the lake or beach like many of our friends, but instead to build our second home at the farm.

The Mysterious Fatigue

With this as a backdrop—my full life that required considerable energy from me as fuel—I was both puzzled and a bit inconvenienced in February 1994 when I experienced this sudden loss of energy. It was an unusual feeling, something I'd never experienced before. It was a kind of all-consuming fatigue, making me feel weak as well as tired. I now call it the "MG feeling."

Initially I passed off the fatigue as being a "low" after being on a "high." We had just experienced a wonderful high in our family—a blessed event, the birth of our first grandchild. Matthew Thomas Powell was born January 10, 1994, to our eldest child, daughter Dr. Rhonda Henderson Powell (OB-GYN), and her husband, Dr. Thomas Powell (orthopedist). Naturally I had been very excited. Aware that I had experienced occasions in my past when I felt a brief "dip" after being up on the mountain emotionally, I thought my fatigue was just a letdown following the excitement of Matthew's birth.

February 1994 also was an especially busy time for MediSphere. We took in more investor money, the structure of our board changed, and I was meeting right and left with doctors who wanted to know more about the company.

After I experienced fatigue for a period in February, the feeling seemed to go away for the most part. Soon thereafter the mysterious fatigue returned. Then it got somewhat better, although I didn't return to my full normal strength. That inexplicable and frustrating pattern continued.

The mysterious fatigue came back, and back, and back. Those periods when I felt considerably below par became longer and more intense.

Even though I was aware this reduced stamina was far from normal for me and was something that had never happened to me before, I didn't go see a physician about it. The reason was that I have always had the philosophy that an individual ought to be able to work through life's challenges and figure out solutions. So I searched for my own solutions.

My solutions soon involved taking steps with which I had no experience—such as setting limits on my schedule in order to conserve my diminishing supply of energy.

Imposing Self-Limits on a Busy Life

I began making adjustments in my usually regimented schedule that I did not like to make. I told myself that the increasing potential and demands of MediSphere was the key reason. But deep down I knew this mysterious fatigue was the tremendous driving factor.

As difficult as it was, I began limiting the number of patients I saw.

Then, something unheard of for me, I began having to take a rest period during the morning, in addition to the afternoon "power nap" I had always taken after I finished my surgery schedule.

Beth and I began cutting out virtually all our social activities because I simply did not have enough stamina.

My regular daily exercising routine also suffered. Exercise is a passion for me, an energizer, something I view as a necessary daily habit for a healthy lifestyle. In early 1994, I had a personal trainer who came to my home daily at 4:30 a.m. to coach me through an hour of programmed exercise—weight-lifting and aerobics—before I went to work. The fatigue became so bad I had to stop that, too.

Time for Major Decisions

In light of all these limitations, I was having to implement changes in my lifestyle to conserve my increasingly declining pool of energy. I was well aware in mid-1994 that I was headed for some real crossroads decisions.

I knew the place where I would go to do that crucial thinking—to my family homeplace near Prattville, on the property of the little farm where I grew up, a few miles from Twin Valley Farms. Each year it was a ritual for me to set aside time to return to my childhood home to contemplate, to reflect in solitude. While going through this process each year, I would accomplish some serious personal and professional planning and goal-setting.

It was in the summer of 1994 when I went to the Henderson homeplace to reflect and plan. By that time I was so energy-deficient I knew I had to consider an option that for me was virtually unthinkable—to give up my practice of medicine. It was a sobering possibility. I loved taking care of patients. I was bonded with my patients. And I was still young in terms of the career-span for a physician, still in my prime—having turned 57 in July 1994. Yet I came to the wrenching conclusion that, in light of this loss of energy I was experiencing, I just did not have the stamina to handle both my medical practice and MediSphere.

Within weeks after that pivotal decision-making trip to my homeplace, I decided to go an agonizing step further: I made the decision that I couldn't even continue personally handling my responsibility as the CEO for Henderson & Walton Women's Center.

A Sad Farewell to Patients

In November 1994, my reluctant retirement from the practice of medicine took on an official tone with a going-away tea for me, an event hosted by my medical partners and held at the beautiful Botanical Gardens in Birmingham.

My fellow physicians at Henderson & Walton Women's Center wanted to do this for me. They also felt we should do it for my patients—especially in light of the kind of response I had been getting from patients when I told them I was retiring. So many of my patients felt like I was abandoning them; they felt I was too young to retire. My retirement was such an abrupt and unexpected announcement. The common theme I heard from patients was, "What am I going to do without you?"

I wish I could say that I recall my goodbye retirement tea as a happy event. I don't. I recall it as more analogous to a wake than to a happy event. We certainly didn't have a problem with lack of turnout for the event. Quite the opposite. We had so many people they had to stop traffic outside, and some 650 signed a guest book and many didn't get around to signing it. But the tea proved to be such an incredibly sad occasion. During the afternoon, I greeted one patient after another as they shared poignant memories of my taking care of them over the years. Since the patients didn't want me to go, and I didn't want to go, they were crying; and I, too, was very emotional. My attorney daughter, Ellen, arrived at the event a little late due to some commitments she had with her law practice. By the time she got there, the line of people waiting to see me had become very long. The tears also were flowing freely. After Ellen arrived and took in what all was going on, she went to find Beth, who was downstairs where people were arriving. She said, "Mom, you've got to go up and rescue Dad. It looks like a wake up there!"

In addition to the in-person contact with those hundreds of patients at the going-away tea, I took home with me two books of my patients' written memories and well-wishes, which Henderson & Walton Women's Center presented to me. These memory books had been put together for my retirement by my executive assistant, Carol Zassoda. Carol had taken the initiative to contact my long-term patients and ask them to write their memories of having me as their doctor. Well, here I had all these wonderful written messages. The patients wrote to me about my relationship with them and their babies—with their entire families for that matter—about going through their joys and sorrows with them. It was so hard for me to read those messages; it still is. I just did not want to leave my patients at that particular point in my life. It was too soon. If I had felt well enough physically to stay, I would have. I would try to read those messages, and it would break my heart. There they were telling me what I had meant to them, and I felt that they had given me so much more than I ever could give them.

I'll have to say that the period surrounding my retirement from medical practice was very painful for me. Being forced out of my practice by this unexplained fatigue was a real blow. For several weeks after the goodbye tea I just went into the tank emotionally.

Changing Gears

Since I had tremendous responsibility riding on my shoulders with MediSphere, I re-energized myself and entered the year 1995 focusing all my professional attention in that direction.

I was helped along in my transition by the fact that for the first several weeks of 1995 my MediSphere office continued to be just upstairs from the Henderson & Walton Women's Center—the OB-GYN center that I had led so long and that I loved so much. This meant I was able to gradually wean myself from those familiar surroundings. Once or twice a day in early 1995, I would drop by the center for a few minutes and visit with former colleagues and express a social greeting to a few patients. That way, for a short period of time I received what I called my "clinical transfusions."

Then, as difficult as it was to leave that environment, when we moved MediSphere's offices to a more business-oriented building in the spring of 1995, the move and the new business environment actually served to give me more energy. Also, I was excited about MediSphere. I felt MediSphere had a model strong enough to make the company a long-term player. I had surrounded myself in MediSphere with some bright, knowledgeable people I had been fortunate to recruit. I felt we were in a good position with our combined knowledge and experience and, most of all, our understanding of healthcare. We had extensive expertise in building infrastructure, utilizing mass purchasing, streamlining office management, and facilitating growth of practices.

I was busy. MediSphere's weekly management team meeting spawned additional meetings with my vice presidents on a staggered basis. I was working the telephones and traveling, mostly in my plane.

However, that mysterious come-and-go fatigue was still there haunting me, and on many days I felt it imposing severe limitations.

Family Crisis

Even when you're feeling tired and low, as I was, you have to realize that life continues to go on around you and that your friends and loved ones have their issues, too.

I am proud to say that our family is a very close family. We reach out to support one another. During the first week of March 1995 our family entered into a very stressful period. I'm just so grateful that, even though my own physical condition was deteriorating, I still was functioning well enough to reach out as a supporter.

This family crisis involved the health of the youngest of our three children, our only son, Bill. It also involved the health of Bill's wife and baby.

Like me, Bill generally had always been healthy. It was unusual for him to become ill. Also like me, Bill was working at a fast pace. He was one of those bright, talented young people working with me at MediSphere, as vice president of development. Bill was in that position not because he was my son. He had earned the position because of his education and experience, his incredible people skills and team-building ability, and his entrepreneurial streak.

As I look back, I think Bill was doing some heavy worrying about some loved ones in early 1995, and I think the stress of those worries could have contributed to his own health problems. For one thing, he had been very concerned about his wife and their unborn child. His wife, Lyn, who had been experiencing complications with her first pregnancy, was nearing the end of her seventh month and had been confined to total bed rest. Also, I'm sure that Bill was doing some worrying about me and my health. After all, Bill worked with me at MediSphere. No matter how little I said about how I felt, Bill is a bright guy and observed for himself a lot of what was going on with me.

What happened was that Bill came down with a flu-like virus that set the stage for him to have Guillain-Barré syndrome—a disorder in which the body's immune system attacks part of the peripheral nervous system. The symptoms can range from weakness and tingling all the way to paralysis; some patients have to be put on a ventilator to breathe. Although this autoimmune disorder occurs rarely, Guillain-Barré can be extremely serious. When it does occur, it's not unusual for it to strike a patient who, like Bill, has just suffered some kind of respiratory or gastrointestinal virus. It also happens occasionally to patients who recently have undergone surgery or have had some kind of vaccination. Some patients like Bill are lucky and overcome it totally. Others are not so lucky and are left with long-lasting, even permanent, weakness or varying degrees of paralysis.

On the morning Bill became very sick with Guillain-Barré, I was aware he had been under the weather with flu-like symptoms. But I was not aware his condition had suddenly deteriorated and taken on additional symptoms. I was sitting in my MediSphere office when I received a phone call from Beth about our son. She said, "You need to go check on Bill. I just talked with him on the phone, and he sounded terrible!" When I walked into Bill's office, I saw immediately that his mother had been correct. Bill was sitting at his desk, with his head down on the desk, very ill. As I stood there and talked with him, the paralysis was apparent. I knew immediately that Bill had Guillain-Barré. His symptoms were classic, and his having had the flu-like illness to set the stage was like being straight out of a medical textbook. I had him hospitalized immediately at the Birmingham hospital where I had practiced all those years, St. Vincent's. Although Bill did not end up on the ventilator and ultimately recovered totally with no aftereffects, he had to have immunoglobulin treatments over about a two-week period.

When Bill got sick, other challenges also came to our family. As fate would have it, within the span of a few hours several things occurred: Bill was admitted to the hospital; our daughter-in-law, Lyn, went into premature labor; and their daughter, Lauren Elise, our second grandchild, was delivered five weeks prematurely—all bang, bang, bang! All three members of that little family were in the same hospital at the same time.

All three ultimately did well—new dad, new mom, and new baby girl. The story had a happy ending. However, it was a stressful time.

Fatigue Becomes a Barometer

As sunshine, clear skies, lush green trees, and colorful flowers ushered in Springtime 1995 to the lovely South where we live, I'll have to say my own state of well-being often was a bleak contrast to the sunny outdoors.

My unexplained physical symptoms were placing my personal and professional life on a dizzying up-and-down rollercoaster.

Often on a given day it was the amount of fatigue that I was feeling, and not other issues, that was determining whether that day proved to be uplifting or stressful, happy or worrisome, productive or compromised, energizing or tiring. To slightly modify the words of a familiar song, "some days were diamonds, but *many* days were stones." This bizarre fatigue clearly was climbing into the driver's seat of my life.

Routine Visit to the Doctor

As the fatigue and weakness had persisted and intensified through the weeks and months, I refrained from picking up the phone to schedule a special appointment with my doctor to make an issue of it. I just kept hoping it would go away.

Then, in the spring of 1995, it was time for my routine annual visit to my internist, my primary-care doctor. This is a doctor's visit that I jokingly have referred to over the years in my OB-GYN lingo as "my annual exam-and-Pap-smear visit."

During that visit, I did tell my physician, Dr. J. Terrell Spencer, that I had been feeling unusually fatigued. However, I didn't make a real big deal out of it to him. I had refused to make a big deal of it to myself. I hadn't even been telling my family how low I had been feeling.

All the time I sat in Terrell's office and talked with him about my fatigue and loss of stamina, I was so cautious about how I presented what I was telling him. After all, there couldn't be anything wrong with me. I had to run MediSphere. I know I was not as honest with him as I should have been. I clearly was in denial.

Terrell and I were doctor and patient; we also were friends. He was familiar with the pace I kept. He knew my work schedule; he knew all the things going on with me professionally. Terrell listened carefully to what I told him; he told me he thought that it was just chronic fatigue and I needed to slow down. Based on how low-key I played this, that was a logical conclusion.

The Road Gets Rockier

The deeper I got into the year 1995, the less my body was cooperating with the pace I was trying to keep. The pattern of fatigue and weakness was getting worse. With my personality and my previous energy level, it was very frustrating to me not to be able to do the things I'd always been able to do ten-fold.

There were days when my fatigue was overwhelming, consuming—days when I would feel totally demoralized. I woke up tired. As the day progressed I became weaker. I went to bed tired. Then I woke up and the tiredness started all over again. The kind of fatigue I had was far beyond the feeling of being physically tired from something like an athletic event or a long day of work. Back in high school, after competing in even the most rigorous football game, I never felt anything close to this fatigue. And prior to having this mysterious fatigue grip me, even my most intense physician-days of seeing patients and performing surgery had never left me this exhausted.

There was no question my strange symptoms were escalating. I began experiencing extreme weakness that seemed to be concentrating, or pooling, in certain parts of my body—weakness that severely limited my ability to use those parts of my body.

For one thing, I started having trouble with a part of me that was my stock and trade—my voice. Usually strong, forceful, and upbeat, my voice was now periodically weak, thin, often raspy or cracking, seldom capable of enduring or projecting, and at times simply giving way. I always had prided myself on being a people person, and I routinely placed a heavy load on my voice in both professional and personal settings. I thrived on conversation and loved to give public speeches. Over the years, I had driven toward many of my business goals via my one-on-one conversations and my speeches to target audiences. With MediSphere, I needed my voice in the worst way. But in the spring, summer, and fall of 1995 my voice often wasn't there for me. Many days I would start losing my voice by 10 o'clock in the morning. If I had to make a speech that evening there was no way to hear me without a microphone, and sometimes it was tough even with a mike's help.

Something also was wrong with my grip and strength. I was having trouble with tasks such as twisting a cap off a bottle and buttoning and unbuttoning my shirts. Picking up anything of any weight was becoming more and more of a chore. This was an abrupt departure from the Ron Henderson of days gone by. I had been the strong farm boy, capable of doing whatever needed to be done on a farm. I had become an adult who excelled with weight-resistant exercising. Now I found myself having trouble trying to lift a suitcase or a bag of garbage. Beth stopped asking me to help her twist off a stubborn bottle cap or to take out the garbage.

Also, I no longer could be sure I could even hold my head up. My neck muscles suddenly would be so weak they couldn't hold my head upright. This tended to happen particularly in the afternoon. I would be in a meeting with someone; I would just be sitting there either talking or listening, and all of a sudden my head would just fall backward!

Covering Up

Even though I was all too aware that something was wrong with me, I didn't want those around me to know. After things got really bad, I did confide to an extent in a limited few from whom I could not hide my symptoms—my beloved wife, Beth; my former medical partner, Dr. Phil Walton; and Belinda Cornelius, the chief operating officer at MediSphere.

But for the most part, for most of the world, I put on an act, a show, to cover up what was going on with me. Unless someone said or asked something direct and pointed about my health status, I didn't bring it up. I was my usual upbeat self. Someone would say, "Ron, how are you doing?" Even if I felt lousy, I would say, "Great!"

I had quick answers when specific questions did come.

When my voice was raspy, if a person would say, "Ron, you sound hoarse," I would reply with something like, "Well, I think I do have a little cold, a little allergy." (This was really good acting! For even though I didn't yet know what was really wrong with my voice, I had lost all reason to hope it was something minor or temporary such as a cold or allergy.)

I even covered up quickly for that disturbing, embarrassing problem of my head just flopping back suddenly. The first time my neck muscles became so weak that I lost control of my head movement was during a meeting at MediSphere on an afternoon in the summer of 1995. I was with a group and we were discussing something, and all of a sudden my head fell back. For me that was a real wake-up moment! But to the others in the room I just kept going forward with the meeting. Since I could not assure myself that my head wouldn't fall back again, I just finished the meeting by cupping my hands underneath my chin to support my head and leaned forward intently to listen and talk.

Maybe I should have gone into acting?

The Self-Diagnosis

In the summer of 1995 I was feeling so terrible that I began studying the scientific literature, searching for an answer to what was wrong with me.

By this time, I was convinced I had a neurological disease. I just didn't know what it was. I knew that something was wrong with my grip, something was wrong with my strength, and a lot was wrong with my stamina.

I also had begun having the symptom of muscle twitching, or fasciculation. That was one of the symptoms of a much-dreaded neurological disease known as "ALS," or amyotrophic lateral sclerosis.

So I added up all my symptoms and made a self-diagnosis.

On Labor Day weekend 1995, while our immediate family was gathered for the holiday at our farm home at Twin Valley, after lunch I called together all the adult members of the family. In a very emotional meeting, I announced to them my self-diagnosis: "I have ALS."

Now, people have a right to be devastated when hearing a diagnosis of ALS associated with themselves or loved ones. Several decades ago this whole nation started becoming familiar with the horror of ALS when this vicious neurological disease ravaged the body of beloved New York Yankees star Lou Gehrig. After ALS claimed the life of Lou Gehrig in 1941, when he was only 37 years old, ALS came to be known to many as "Lou Gehrig's Disease." This is an always-fatal disease in which the voluntary muscles of the body waste away rapidly because of an attack on the nerve cells that control these muscles. In addition to the wasting away, the atrophy, there is also considerable muscle twitching, or fasciculation. Most patients are dead within three to five years following diagnosis, some much sooner. In the course of dying, the victims become unable to move their arms, legs, and other parts of the body, and ultimately are unable to breathe.

Thank goodness I would prove to be wrong in my self-diagnosis.

I must say here that any doctor who self-diagnoses is a fool, and any doctor who treats himself is a fool. That takes all the objectivity out of the process. I have no one to blame except myself that I made this incorrect self-diagnosis. For that matter, I have no one to blame except myself that I focused my attention on finding a diagnosis myself instead of being more honest about my symptoms and more aggressive in my search for a diagnosis from other physicians.

The way I had arrived at my self-diagnosis was reviewing the neurological-diseases literature and methodically going through a "differential diagnosis" process—matching my own symptoms with various diagnoses to rule out this or that, or to rule in this or that. The symptoms I was having were not a good match for several neurological diseases, including multiple sclerosis. As it turned out, my clinical picture was also not a real good match for ALS, but at the time the fact I was having the muscle twitching really convinced me.

Making this grim ALS announcement was a terrible thing to do to my family—to my wife, three children, and son-in-law and daughter-in-law. Even though it was an emotional experience making that announcement, my family members are savvy, strong people; and they handled it well. At least, they handled it well in my presence. Keep in mind that my family members who faced me in the room that day all had considerable exposure to the healthcare world. They included the longtime wife of a physician who also was a central caregiver in her family, two medical doctors, a registered nurse, a business professional who had worked for years in the health field, and an attorney with a client base that included a lot of doctors.

A driving force in my decision to reveal my ALS self-diagnosis to my family members was that I *had* to talk to them candidly. While I was covering up my health problems with many people, I had come to the point I felt compelled to discuss my health situation openly with members of my family. They knew I was down. I couldn't hide that from them. They knew I was not as interactive with them, that I was spending a lot of time in bed when I was home.

The same day I made my ALS announcement to members of my family I also informed them of my intentions as far as what I planned to do next. I told them I was determined to continue to live my life as normally and as fully as possible, for as long as possible—which with ALS likely would not be long at all. I said, "I'm going to go as far as I can."

The Real Diagnosis

Just as I told my family I planned to do, I did keep going. I continued to work. I did not go to a physician to confirm my self-diagnosis.

Then, two and a half months after I had announced my self-diagnosis to my family, one night in mid-November 1995 I had reason to rethink the diagnostic conclusion I had reached.

On that November evening, I had just returned to Birmingham from a MediSphere business trip to Raleigh, North Carolina. It had been a quick trip, and a busy one. I had traveled alone in my plane. While I was there, my main mission was to make a two-hour presentation on MediSphere to a group of internal medicine specialists who were looking for a PPM company such as ours with which to affiliate.

The two-and-a-half hour plane trip home was not one of my more relaxed flights. I encountered bad weather, and I had to do some maneuvering around thunderstorms. Just east of Atlanta I had to deal with a huge thunderstorm.

By the time I reached home, I was very fatigued. So I rested while Beth finished up dinner. She prepared a steak that night, and I sat down at the dinner table with her looking forward to enjoying our steak dinner. However, as I tried to chew the meat I ran into problems. I simply could not chew efficiently. I knew that another symptom was now rearing its head for the first time—weakness in my muscles of mastication, or chewing.

My brain spun into overdrive trying to process all this. This chewing thing was a real tip-off. Within seconds I knew.

I had been reading so much about neurological diseases that I was aware in ALS the victim's swallowing muscles tend to collapse first and that an ALS patient's chewing muscles are affected after the loss of the ability to swallow.

Well, I could still swallow.

Also from my reading I had expanded my knowledge about a certain neurological disease in which it's common for the chewing muscles to be affected when a patient is still able to swallow. As my brain recalled what I knew about that disease, my symptoms began lining up as a match.

I looked across the table at Beth and said, "Darling, I have some good news and some bad news."

She raised her eyebrows and gave me that intent, questioning look of hers.

"The good news, Beth, is that I don't have ALS. The bad news is that I do have myasthenia gravis."

This time, I did telephone a neurologist to review my suspicions. I called Dr. David O'Neal, and the next morning I was in his office. David ordered two hours of testing on me. That included the diagnostic test using the chemical Tensilon®, to which I had a positive response. When a patient with myasthenia gravis-like symptoms is exposed to Tensilon® and symptoms improve significantly, albeit temporarily, that's a strong clue pointing toward a myasthenia gravis diagnosis.

It didn't take Dr. David O'Neal long to confirm my diagnosis.

I had myasthenia gravis.

2

GETTING FAMILIAR
WITH MYASTHENIA GRAVIS

Now that I had a diagnosis to explain what was wrong with me, I was anxious to learn as much as I could about this rare disease called myasthenia gravis, or MG.

When I was diagnosed in November 1995, I knew I had to take immediate steps to become an expert on MG in order to assume as much control as possible over my destiny with this disease. I believe that's true for all patients who have MG, or who have any other chronic disease for that matter.

By the time I was diagnosed, I already knew a good bit about MG. I had learned a little about it in medical school—*very* little, because very little is taught about it in medical school. Then I had picked up a little additional MG information here and there during my almost three decades of practicing medicine (two years as a family doctor and 26 years as a specialist in OB-GYN). However, I had never had a patient who had MG. There was no doubt that I had accumulated the majority of my MG knowledge during recent months. I had gained knowledge about MG while I was researching various neurological diseases, in my effort to identify what was attacking my own body and sapping my strength and energy.

After I was diagnosed, I felt my background as a doctor would give me an edge in understanding MG. At the same time, I strongly felt that nothing could give me as much of an edge as just being a MG patient and experiencing the symptoms firsthand.

As I sat in my neurologist's office in November 1995 with the new knowledge that myasthenia gravis now was officially a part of my life, I

put my mind in gear to become quickly and deeply familiar with myasthenia gravis. I began going over truths I knew about this disease—truths
I would expand and clarify in weeks and months to come:

• **The disease deserves the literal meaning of its name.** The term "myasthenia gravis" is Latin and Greek in origin, and it means "grave muscle
weakness." After having lived with untreated symptoms for 21 months,
I could vouch firsthand that there was a fit between the disease and the
"grave muscle weakness" label.

• **MG is rare. I was not going to find huge numbers of fellow patients
with this disease.** Having MG is not like having heart disease or arthritis
or one of the major cancers—conditions or diseases that affect many
people. According to the Myasthenia Gravis Foundation of America,
Inc., (MGFA) there are only about 14 individuals per 100,000 population in this nation who have been diagnosed with MG. (There is no hard
data to support this statistic.) Even though MG is hard to diagnose and
experts speculate there are many undiagnosed cases out there, there's no
doubt the disease still would be rare even if all the undiagnosed cases
were uncovered.

• **It's hard to diagnose MG, and more often than not there is a major
delay in diagnosis.** I know I likely delayed my own diagnosis by trying
to diagnose myself—far from an objective process. However, while it was
21 months from my first symptoms to diagnosis, the National Institutes
of Health reports it's not unusual for a patient to experience a year to two
years of delay in having his or her MG diagnosed. For many patients,
that agonizing waiting period is even longer. Some MGFA chapters have
members who searched for a diagnosis *for several years.* Among those are
many patients—especially female patients—who were told by their doctors that they should see psychiatrists because they were just imagining
the symptoms. Obviously, there's a big need for more MG education in
both the consumer and the medical community. One reason MG is so
hard to diagnose is that this disease really is complex, in that the symp-

toms can appear in different parts of the body and often not seem to be related as components of a central diagnosis. However, another reason MG is so hard to diagnose is that there's a lack of education about this disease among doctors. Many doctors have never been taught to be alert to the possibility that these diverse symptoms could indeed be related and could add up to MG.

• **Although all cases of MG involve symptoms of muscle weakness, these symptoms can affect patients in different ways.** This means that from patient to patient the MG symptoms can affect muscles in different parts of the body, and the MG symptoms can attack patients with varying degrees of severity. Basically, MG is a disease in which there is weakness and loss of control and strength in various voluntary muscle groups in the body. The muscle groups commonly affected are the muscles of the eyes, face, shoulder, and hip and those muscles related to chewing and swallowing. But it doesn't have to stop there; other body muscles could be affected as well. If you have MG, you could have the drooping eyelids, double vision, slurred speech or nasal quality to speech, problems chewing and/or swallowing, choking episodes, trouble holding your head erect, trouble walking or gripping or lifting, general muscle fatigue, various combinations of those, and even additional symptoms. You can suffer life-threatening symptoms—such as weakness of your breathing muscles that could place you on life support, or weakness of your swallowing muscles that could cause you to choke. You can have what is known as generalized or systemic MG, which affects various parts of your body. On the other hand, you can have a more localized form of MG that affects only your eyes. Many MG patients have this localized eye version of the disease. It's appropriately called "ocular MG," and all the MG symptoms are confined to the eye areas—trouble with eye movements, double vision, drooping eyelids, or a combination thereof. I was not one of those to suffer from the localized form. I have generalized or systemic MG—meaning the disease affects muscle groups in various parts of my body.

• **In terms of placing MG in a category relevant to the parts of the body that it affects, MG is what's known as a "neuromuscular disease."** MG is a disease in which the messages don't get from the nerves to the muscles to make the muscles contract as they should.

• **In terms of placing MG in a category relevant to where the disease-causing enemy lives, MG is an "autoimmune disease."** This means MG is one of those diseases in which the patient's own immune system turns on the patient. The enemy causing the disease is not some outside virus or bacteria that invades the patient's body; instead, the enemy lives inside the patient's own body. If a person has an autoimmune disease, this means he has a disease in which his own antibodies in some way are waging war on his body's own molecules, cells, or tissues. There are several diseases in this category—including multiple sclerosis, Guillain-Barré syndrome, type I diabetes (formerly known as juvenile diabetes), lupus (technically called SLE or systemic lupus erythematosus), and rheumatoid arthritis. Obviously if we can learn more about MG, it likely can help us wage war on some or all of these other autoimmune diseases.

• **The autoimmune war being waged in MG involves antibodies forming in the MG patient's body and causing destruction of important "receptor sites" that play a key role in making the muscles contract.** The job of making the muscles contract involves roles played by both the body's nerve endings and the muscle fibers. Vital activity that triggers the muscle contraction takes place at the junction, or space, between where the nerve endings and the muscle fibers come together—an area appropriately called the "neuromuscular junction." Playing a big part in making muscles contract are receptor sites known as acetylcholine receptors, or AChR. Normally, the muscles contract when these receptor sites have been activated by a chemical that gives the receptor sites their name—the chemical known as acetylcholine. In keeping with the close relationship between the nerve endings and the muscles, the acetylcholine chemical is released on the nerve ending side of the neuromuscular junction, and the chemical travels across the junction to bind with the AChR sites that are located on the muscle fiber side of the junction. However, for some reason not clearly understood, some of the myasthenia gravis patient's AChR sites are being altered, blocked, and/or destroyed by abnormal antibodies being produced in the patient's own immune system. Since the MG patient has fewer healthy receptor sites to be activated by the acetylcholine, the patient suffers resulting muscle-weakness problems. This includes weakness, fatigue, and loss of strength and function in whatever voluntary muscles that happen to be affected in a given MG patient. The locations of those muscles and how badly they are affected can vary greatly from one MG patient to another.

• **There is no explanation for why a particular individual gets MG.** It just happens. MG is not contagious. There's no solid evidence MG is inherited, although there might be genetic trends or patterns. (I have firm reason to believe there likely are genetic "patterns" at play in some cases, including my own case. Another rare neurological disorder that's a close MG relative—a disorder called Guillain-Barré syndrome—has stricken two immediate members of my family. Those family members are my son, Bill, and my younger brother, Tommy.) I'm more than slightly interested in learning more about the possible genetic patterns.

• **Back in 1995 when I was diagnosed, one of the most important things I understood about MG was that it is a chronic, incurable disease.** The disease wasn't likely to be temporary, wasn't likely to go away. MG was not a short-term health problem for which I could go to my doctor and get a prescription, visit my druggist and get the prescription filled, take pills for a few days, and get well. Unless a cure could be found, I knew I likely would be living with this chronic disease for the rest of my life. I knew I had reason to embrace a tiny hope that I would be one of the fortunate MG patients to enjoy a "remission"—in which the MG symptoms just disappear for a time, or maybe indefinitely. I knew that this remission miracle occasionally occurs even with some patients like me who have the more severe generalized, systemic form of MG. However, I also knew I would be in the minority if this were to happen, because most of the MG patients who enjoy a remission tend to be those with the localized "ocular MG." Thus I prepared to approach my disease for the long haul. I knew that for the foreseeable future all that could be done for my MG would be to use treatments to control the disease's symptoms. The treatments that work for one patient might not work for another. Each MG patient needs tailored treatment. I knew that, just like a patient with any chronic disease, I now had to work with my doctors in managing my disease. So, beginning in November 1995, I started learning to live with this chronic, neuromuscular, autoimmune disease called myasthenia gravis.

3

Confronting the Realities of Myasthenia Gravis

When I left the office of neurologist Dr. David O'Neal on that day I was diagnosed in November 1995, I knew I had to go forward and wage two battles simultaneously. One battle was to reclaim as much of my health as possible by dealing effectively with the myasthenia gravis. The other battle was in the business world, in my role as CEO of MediSphere.

I still had high hopes for the success of MediSphere. However, I rapidly was reaching the conclusion that I should make arrangements for someone besides me to be at MediSphere's helm. Even though I now had a diagnosis of what was wrong with me and would be on treatments to control the MG symptoms, I knew that even under the best scenario it likely would take awhile to get my MG stabilized. And, even if and when my condition was stabilized, I had no way of predicting how close to full strength and stamina I would be. MediSphere was a high-pressure, fast-paced start-up company. I felt the company needed someone at the helm who had a consistent supply of abundant, predictable energy and stamina.

So, soon after my diagnosis, I began to focus my attention on two parallel tracks where MediSphere was concerned. At the same time I would work especially hard to "grow" the company, I was going to search for a new caretaker or new partner for the company. That meant finding someone else to run MediSphere, including perhaps going as far as a merger.

Little could I envision the horrendous MediSphere business perils that lay ahead during the next 15 pressure-filled months.

Keeping My Diagnosis in the Closet

Once I knew about my diagnosis, I initially shared that information with as few people as possible. I told only those I felt really needed to know. I wanted that information to be placed in a special closet, and only a few family members, friends, and business associates to have the keys to the closet.

I had a heartfelt personal reason that was a motivator to keep my MG diagnosis secret from most of those around me. The reason was that I did not want word of my diagnosis to reach the ears of my mother or Beth's mother. I felt this news would be devastating to both of those women, who were up in years and very much a part of my life. I had a close relationship with both of them. Beth and I were the primary caregivers for her mother. And for my mother I was her first line for everything. Both of my brothers lived out of state, and I was the one to whom my mother turned for her day-to-day needs.

There were other reasons why I didn't want to go around telling everyone I had MG.

The well-being of MediSphere was a major reason. I feared the impact that widespread knowledge of my diagnosis might have on the company and on physicians and employees whose livelihoods were dependent on MediSphere.

Too, I didn't want to be treated "differently" by other people. I wanted people to react to me as one who is strong, in control, and positive, the same way they always had reacted to me. I didn't want people to see me as compromised in any way. Being viewed as somewhat compromised is one negative image likely to confront many an individual suffering from a chronic disease.

So, as I shared my MG news with a chosen few, I accompanied it with my "please do not tell anyone" speech. I told my children and their spouses, "Now, this is a private family matter; and I ask that you please don't discuss it with your friends or other people." I did make the decision to explain my MG diagnosis to all members of my MediSphere executive committee; but I cautioned them that this was in-house company information, not to be shared with others. And of course I shared the news with my longtime friend and former medical partner, Dr. Phil Walton, with whom I knew my secret was safe.

With Mestinon® in Hand

Although there are several approaches that can be used to treat the symptoms of myasthenia gravis, a number of the treatments have extensive side effects and carry long-term risk factors. From the start, I participated with my doctors in decisions about my treatments. I told them that wherever possible I wanted my condition approached with the least drastic interventions.

The first treatment I received for MG was conservative. It involved my taking the prescription medication Mestinon®—with the goal of reducing the amount and severity of the muscle weakness I was feeling. When a patient responds well to Mestinon® treatment, there is less muscle weakness and also much less overall fatigue. The goal of Mestinon® is to increase the ability of the nerves to get information through to tell the muscles to contract. Normally in transmitting this nerve-to-muscle information and triggering muscle contraction in a patient who does not have MG, there's a smooth process by which a chemical called acetylcholine activates some receptors. The activation of these vital receptors by this chemical takes place at the "neuromuscular junction"—a space between where the nerve endings and muscle fibers meet. However, in the patient who has MG, the patient's own immune system is producing antibodies that are destroying or altering the receptors. What Mestinon® does is to make more of the chemical acetylcholine available to this diminished supply of receptors, by preventing the breakdown of acetylcholine and allowing it to accumulate and remain at the neuromuscular junction longer than usual.

Mestinon® can be taken in 60-milligram tablets, 180-milligram long-acting tablets, injectable form, or a syrup version. I started taking Mestinon® by mouth, the tablets, and Dr. O'Neal and I worked on adjusting the dosage. I ended up taking it every three hours during the day, 90 milligrams at a time, and then taking the 180-milligram long-lasting tablet to carry me through the night.

At the beginning, soon after going on Mestinon® and continuing for several months, I began feeling better, stronger. I was especially pleased that Mestinon® brought me considerable relief from a MG symptom that had become a particular problem—the lack of strength and control, and accompanying pain, in my neck muscles.

Then, in the summer of 1996, even the Mestinon® did not keep my MG symptoms at bay. That summer hit me terribly. Actually, even though I'm doing much better as I write this in 2002, I am very aware that I feel noticeably stronger in the spring, fall, and winter than I do in the summer. I've talked to many other MG patients who tell me the same thing—particularly those who, like myself, live in a hot climate. The heat tends to be tough on many myasthenics. And I can tell you that summertime in Alabama can deliver its share of hot, humid days.

After the fall of 1996 brought the cooler weather, I began feeling somewhat better again. However, that didn't last long. The winter of 1996 was not a good one for my MG symptoms. I was not well. (After my condition finally got stabilized, I found that winters tend to be good periods for my MG.)

By late 1996, it was becoming increasingly apparent that, in order to control my MG, the Mestinon® needed some helpmates—help from some of the stronger MG treatments. However, I was reluctant at that point to go through the rigors of those treatments.

In the period immediately following my diagnosis, I was treated by two physicians. My MG condition was treated by Dr. David O'Neal, the neurologist who had diagnosed me. For my general healthcare management, I continued to see my primary-care doctor, Dr. J. Terrell Spencer. Then, at Dr. O'Neal's suggestion, in early 1996 I had added a third doctor. I also began seeing Birmingham neurologist Dr. Shin Oh, whose specialty is myasthenia gravis.

When I initially saw Dr. Oh in early 1996, it was his strong recommendation that I add immunosuppressive drug therapy to my treatment regimen. Dr. Oh recommended that I continue taking the Mestinon® and also add the immunosuppressant drugs prednisone and Imuran®. I resisted. I knew there were long-term risks to immunosuppressants. I knew that prednisone, a steroid medication, could put you at long-term risk for problems such as osteoporosis, diabetes, cataracts, and glaucoma. I knew that Imuran® carried a long-term risk for certain cancers. And just on a day-to-day basis I knew that prednisone could cause side effects that make you jittery, interfere with your sleeping patterns, make you have mood swings, and increase your vulnerability to infections.

So it was in early 1996 that I had decided to go against Dr. Oh's recommendation and to keep trying to manage my MG with Mestinon® alone. There's no doubt I was partly motivated in this decision by what was going on in my business life. I felt that I surely didn't need to take medication that could make me feel jittery and suffer mood swings while I was trying to deal with the mounting business pressures of MediSphere. I wanted to keep my head as clear as possible to guide that company through the much-troubled waters it now was traveling. As 1995 and 1996 wore on, I increasingly knew that with MediSphere I had a tiger by the tail.

Taking Care of MediSphere

At the time I had founded MediSphere in the early 1990s, concepts such as managed care and businesslike approaches to medicine were riding a high crest of popularity and potential. It seemed to be the wave of the future that increasing numbers of doctor groups would link with business companies in a win-win model put forth by this approach labeled "PPM," or physician practice management.

However, by the year 1996 we began to hear loud rumblings of doubt and discontent about the PPM industry's basic business model. Some "doubting Thomases" who voiced concerns to me would praise the strengths of this PPM company known as MediSphere, but in the next breath express skepticism about the long-term viability of the overall PPM concept.

In the mid-1990s, several issues began coming together on a collision course to impact the PPM industry. It seemed like a runaway freight train. One issue, a big one, was the uncertain future of managed care. Another was the unyielding tendency for most American doctors to be autonomy-driven individuals—independent operators who don't engage comfortably or effectively as team players with business companies. Still another, an issue that's been there for centuries and doesn't seem to be improving very fast, is the unwillingness of doctors to change—doctors' tendency not to understand how to bring about good management and not to appreciate the value of good management. In my opinion, the biggest problem that doctors still have today is being tied to the habits of the past.

Added to all this difficult climate in 1996 was the fact that some PPM companies around the nation were running into problems executing the business models they had touted so vocally. In my opinion, some problems faced by certain PPM companies were tied partly to the issues I listed above, while other problems resulted from these companies not generating enough value. I think there were some PPM companies that were entering into business deals with doctor groups and just taking money out of the doctors' practices without returning much value. This would set the stage for major failures of some of these companies in 1997, 1998, and afterward.

Needless to say, this skeptical-of-PPM-companies climate in 1996 was impeding MediSphere's ability to secure the additional funding it needed to move forward. MediSphere had business and the promise of much more business. But in order to take advantage of those business opportunities we needed cash. As changes and concerns mounted in the PPM industry, venture capital companies, private investors, and doctors became increasingly skeptical.

Despite these rocky PPM roads, in 1996 there still were many doctors interested in doing deals with MediSphere—that is, if MediSphere could find the cash to do the deals. In the spring of 1996, MediSphere was attracting so much positive attention and our people in the company were doing such a good job that we had some 200 doctors under letters of intent with MediSphere. These doctors were spread out over several states. To implement these deals, some of the doctor groups wanted all cash, some all stock, some a combination of both. Cash is king when you're a start-up company in a rapid-growth phase like MediSphere was at the time. Cash flow is vital to a start-up company. No matter which way you cut it, we had to have more cash infused into the business.

There had been a time early in MediSphere's development when I had been offered $20 million for 50 percent of MediSphere. Now I was struggling to find investor money to keep the company going. I was out there searching for money at a time when the investor appetite for PPMs had gone sour. During 1996, my MediSphere vice presidents and I talked with one venture capital company after another—probably as many as 20 of them. One of these companies that I particularly recall strung us along for three months, led us to believe we had a deal, and backed out on us at the 11th hour.

While all this was unfolding, I wasn't doing well at all in trying to control my MG symptoms with the help of Mestinon® alone. If stress does aggravate one's health problems, particularly an autoimmune health problem such as MG—and I believe stress indeed is a vicious aggravator, and probably even an initiator—I wasn't doing my health any favors with the stress I was bringing to it via MediSphere.

Beth, my ever-supportive wife, was very concerned about the stress being put on me by the company. She kept telling me that I needed to get out from under this stress, that I needed to find somewhere to put the company.

In the late fall of 1996, it reached the point that I knew MediSphere was looking straight at bankruptcy if we didn't get an infusion of money. I knew if I didn't find some investor money quickly, or if I didn't find a merger deal, we were going to have to shut down MediSphere and I was going to have to let all my wonderful people go in one fell swoop. At the same time, I still was convinced that MediSphere had great potential. I felt if the company could find a viable partner with which to join hands, it still could be a win-win. If that didn't happen . . . Well, I didn't have many options, because I was running out of time.

During that difficult time, I felt a tremendous responsibility to the doctors and the employees who already were associated with MediSphere. This company was my deal, my responsibility; it was on my shoulders. The buck stopped with me. By late 1996, when things became so touch-and-go, we had eight physician practices, in several Southern states, already affiliated with MediSphere. Included in those eight doctor practices were physicians who were my friends. Several of these doctors had known me for many years. One, for example, had been a fellow undergraduate student with me at the University of Alabama, and also had been a fellow medical student and then a fellow intern. Another MediSphere affiliate was a physician who had known me since I was a young family doctor in my 20s practicing in the small town of Gordo, Alabama. While I had practiced in Gordo, this other physician who was now a MediSphere affiliate had practiced in another nearby town.

The cash flow crisis in MediSphere was "coming to a head" so to speak in late 1996 when MediSphere did two major deals, and in order to make those deals happen I had to go on a line of credit personally for $2 million. I always had promised Beth I wouldn't do that, and now being put in a position to have to do it put me under additional stress.

In the meantime, I had met a businessman who was running another PPM company—one based in Nashville, Tennessee. He was interested in MediSphere. The company he headed had money, but it did not have much business. Conversely, MediSphere had many business opportunities, but we were running out of money. This businessman and I began talking merger. Our two companies looked like a perfect fit.

It was December 1996 when we launched serious merger talks. We seemed to be on the same page, and within a short time I thought we had the terms all set. But once we took a term sheet to his company, there were major conflicts as we got into details. Between the time we started putting things together in December and when we consummated the deal a few weeks later in February 1997, we were embroiled in what I would term intense, controversial, brutal negotiations.

However, beginning in February 1997 MediSphere did have a new home. Its headquarters moved to Nashville. The company also had a new name—MediSphere Health Partners, the same name under which the company continues to operate today. For the time being, I would stay on as chairman, but I would be able to relinquish the day-to-day pressure of serving as CEO. In my new role, I would continue living in

Alabama and would fly to Nashville frequently.

As I look back on 1997 in MediSphere—my last year in a high-profile MediSphere role—I think of three words to describe it. Number one, *relief*—relief that the company did have a home and was continuing to function. Number two, *frustration*—frustration because I disagreed with many of the day-to-day decisions and management style approaches that began coming into play soon after the merger was completed. And, thirdly, *turbulence*. The turbulence was there because of internal changes spawned by the merger. The turbulence was there also because of external pressures radiating from highly publicized crises sustained by other PPMs around the nation, such as MedPartners and PhyCor. Although MediSphere Health Partners was surviving, it was not meeting nearly the potential I had envisioned and it was impacted by negative PPM fallout beyond its control. However, I'm just glad that the company has continued to be a survivor.

Taking Drastic Steps To Address MG

By the end of 1997, I was feeling so poorly that I knew I was at another crossroads. I knew my myasthenia gravis condition was out of control, and I knew further that I would have to resort to drastic steps to bring it under control.

I was exhausted both physically and emotionally. In addition to the rigors of MediSphere, the year 1997 had been a sad, difficult one in my personal life. That was the year my mother died.

Two years back, in late 1995 when my MG was diagnosed, I had committed to myself that I would focus on both the health of MediSphere and my own health. Keeping that dual promise proved not to be in the cards. During those first two crucial years that I knew I had MG, it was MediSphere that consumed virtually all my time, energy, and attention. By the end of 1997, I didn't have to have someone tell me that I had been focusing on MediSphere's health at the expense of my own.

Now I had no choice but to change that.

Over the 1997 Christmas holidays, Beth and I made the decision that I would take a six-month sabbatical from MediSphere. By this time, it was common knowledge within the company that I had MG. Thus, my sabbatical came as little surprise to leaders of the company. I had one goal in mind—to free up my time and commitments so that I could devote the attention required to start taking care of my health in earnest.

In mid-February 1998, feeling really in the tank healthwise, I went to see neurologist Dr. Shin Oh. I apologized to Dr. Oh for not going on prednisone and Imuran® two years previously when he first told me I should. I told him I was ready to try it. So two days later we started. Each morning I would take 60 milligrams of prednisone and 150 milligrams of Imuran®.

In addition to the decision Beth and I made that I would take the sabbatical from MediSphere, she and I also made another decision. We decided that, for several months in early 1998, we would not live in Birmingham, that instead we would move to our "second home" at our farm. This move would give me a private place to rest and take my medicines. I would be retreating to the beautiful, secluded site on our Twin Valley Farms property near Prattville, Alabama, about an hour-and-a-half drive south of Birmingham.

One thing I liked about going to the farm was that this would get me away from people while I was taking high dosages of immunosuppressants. While I couldn't predict exactly how the steroids would impact my behavior, I didn't think the impact would be good. Also, I knew these immunosuppressants would make it easy for me to catch contagious illnesses, and I would be at higher risk if I were interacting with large numbers of people.

I said I was going to the farm to get to feeling better. I knew, too, that I was going to the farm to hide.

Dealing with Immunosuppressant Therapy

There's an old saying about having to take the bad with the good. I know that's often true. A lot of times in order to get the benefits of something you have to take the hard knocks that go with it. For me, the initial period of taking those immunosuppressants would be far from a picnic. There would be days when I thought I would climb the walls taking that stuff.

However, I will say this: There is no doubt in my mind that these immunosuppressants did play a significant role in helping me get back on the road toward a healthier life. (I would ultimately get off the Imuran® and drastically reduce the prednisone.) As I look back to the days beginning in early 1998 when I was taking high dosages, I'm grateful for what these medications did for me.

But, wow!! I doubt if any of those around me will soon forget the Ron Henderson who was on the steroid prednisone in the year 1998.

Several years earlier, I had taken a short-lived round of prednisone to treat allergies, and I had not reacted well to the medication. Recalling that experience and also knowing a good deal about steroid medication, Beth and I both expected I would have a rocky course with the prednisone in 1998. Boy, were we ever correct!

You see, one problem with prednisone is that it really can temporarily change your personality. If you're a hyper guy like I am—a hard-driving "type A personality"—steroid medication is especially likely to put you into orbit. Mix my personality with a lot of prednisone, throw in MG, and you can get on a real high. When you drop down, it's really like a crash.

All that is exactly what happened to me. It was really disturbing. To say I had a "rocky course" is an understatement. That prednisone put me above the atmosphere into the stratosphere and then dumped me back again. I went ballistic. Up and down, up and down; again and again. I had insomnia. I was up at 3 to 4 a.m., even earlier that I usually had gotten up in my old days as a doctor. Once I got up, I was so hyper and jittery that I did bizarre things. For instance, I would sit there in the sunroom/den and get on the phone and start ordering things out of catalogs. I would call this nice woman I never met, who was an order clerk for one of these catalog companies. She was a nice lady, but the main thing is that she was awake and was someone to talk to. I'd call her and order something out of the catalog just to have something to do.

Oh, the mood swings I had! The abrupt shifts in energy level! When I got up each morning, even though I had had little sleep I believed I was on top of the mountain, filled with huge amounts of energy that bordered on euphoria. (It was false energy, prednisone energy.) For two or three hours while Beth slept in the wee hours of the morning, I ordered out of the catalog, worked on an outline for a book, read voraciously, and made entries in my daily diary. And then by the time Beth was up and starting her day, I started hitting bottom with mine. I'd be at 30,000 feet at five o'clock in the morning, and below sea level by eight o'clock in the morning. I would be exhausted and would go back to bed.

Many days at the farm during 1998 I spent 20 hours out of 24 in the bed—sometimes sleeping, mostly not, just mostly lying there with that all-engulfing "MG feeling."

There were other days when I managed to muster up enough strength to stay up long enough to give orders and drive everyone around me crazy. I would get huge spurts of energy and come up with project after project to keep everyone else busy. My mind whirled with ideas! I would look out over the farm, the barns, our home, other buildings, and the beef operation; then I would decide we needed to do this and that project. Among projects we implemented during that period was building a guest-house down the hill from our farm home at Twin Valley. Throughout my professional life, it had been my style to delegate extensively. During my intensive prednisone-taking days at Twin Valley, I delegated, delegated, delegated. I would get an idea, tell other people to get it started, go back to bed while they got busy, muster up energy to get up and inspect what they had done, and then start over with more ideas and assignments. I know I drove Beth crazy and drove other members of our family crazy. And I know it had to be maddening for our wonderful Twin Valley Farms cattle manager, Roland Starnes.

On a positive note about the steroids, I succeeded in taking aim at certain potential side effects. The weapon I used was self-discipline. Among prednisone side effects is that it increases your appetite. Many people gain a lot of weight and get the look of being moon-faced. I never got the moon face; maybe that was luck and self-discipline combined. I *know* the lack of weight gain was self-discipline. When I was taking large dosages of prednisone, I got so hungry I could have eaten the paint off the walls! But no matter how hungry I got, I watched what I ate and drank a lot of water. The result was that I gained very little weight.

Two More Health Problems

In 1998, while I was getting adjusted to the immunosuppressant therapy, I encountered two more healthcare challenges with which I would wage an up-and-down battle.

I started having bouts with asthma and bronchitis. Seventeen years prior to that, I had a spell of asthma and bronchitis due to some mold that invaded the downstairs exercise room at our home. I responded to treatment; the asthma and bronchitis went away.

Now they had returned. Most of the time when I got a cold, the asthma and bronchitis seemed to follow. And after I went on immuno-suppressants I got one cold after another.

There's no way for me to know if there was a connection between the bronchitis and asthma and my immune system being suppressed by the prednisone and the Imuran®. It's possible there was just a trade-off.

I also began searching the literature trying to figure out the relation-ship between asthma, bronchitis, and myasthenia gravis. It's commonly known that asthma and MG both are autoimmune diseases. But in the literature they're not connected.

I do know that I'm not the only one in the family who has had trouble with asthma. Our grandson, Matthew, has severe asthma episodes. Our oldest granddaughter, Lauren, also has asthma. I'm beginning to believe more and more in genetic patterns, trends, connections, and predisposi-tions with autoimmune problems. Matthew, Lauren, and I have asthma, an autoimmune disorder. I have myasthenia gravis, an autoimmune disease. And my son, Bill, and my youngest brother, Tommy, both have suffered from the same rare autoimmune disorder, Guillain-Barré syndrome.

Slow Response to the Immunosuppressants

The reason a MG patient takes prednisone and Imuran® is to ma-nipulate the immune system. These immunosuppressant medications are some of the same ones that have been used over the years to manipulate the immune systems of organ transplant patients, to prevent them from rejecting their transplanted organs.

If you're a MG patient whose doctor has recommended these medications, the goal is to suppress your immune system so that you don't build up certain antibodies. After all, MG is an autoimmune disease in which your body is building antibodies that are interfering with the function of your muscles. In a myasthenic patient, the immune system is overactive and the goal of immunosuppressants is to suppress that overactivity.

Generally speaking, taking both prednisone and Imuran® together can bring about miraculous effects for some MG patients. However, about the earliest you can expect any major improvement is three months to a year after you start taking the medications. It especially takes a long time for Imuran® to be effective.

For me, it took much longer than average before I really felt a bang for the buck with the Imuran® and prednisone. Actually, it took about 15 months. It was well into the year 2000—around May or June of 2000—before I began to feel noticeably and significantly better. But, thank goodness, that time finally arrived.

The reason for the delay in my reaping treatment benefits is simple: Generally, the longer you've had MG, the longer it's likely to take for immunosuppressant therapy such as prednisone and Imuran® to help you. There seems to be a direct relationship.

Thus, the way I look at it I paid this price of experiencing a long delay in enjoying treatment benefits because I repeatedly had delayed addressing my MG. First, I had delayed seeking help from physicians in getting a diagnosis and instead had tried to diagnose myself. Then, after I was diagnosed, for two years I focused on taking care of MediSphere in a stressful, pressure-cooker environment instead of taking care of myself. (I look back, and I still don't know how I could have done otherwise with MediSphere. I could not desert that company!) But, right or wrong, preventable or unpreventable, the fact remains that exactly four years elapsed from the time I felt my first symptoms, in February 1994, until I started on immunosuppressant therapy in February 1998. Included in all this was my two-year delay from the time Dr. Shin Oh recommended immunosuppressant therapy until I started it.

I'm just grateful to my doctors for hanging in there with me, for working with me to overcome the problems I had caused with these delays.

Missing the Activity and Camaraderie

It's not easy for *anyone* to be sick and then to become isolated from much of the outside world because of that sickness. However, I think some people do better with it than others.

Over the years, in my experience as a physician and also as a friend to many hard-driving people like me, I have found that people like me are among those who have the most difficult times with being sick and isolated.

These people to whom I refer are those who are high-energy, have many balls in the air, display driven type A personality traits, are accustomed to holding leadership roles and being in charge, are restless and creative and always involved in new projects, and thrive on interaction with people.

I had never planned to feel old and certainly not to get sick. My entire lifestyle had been centered around activities designed to maintain good health and increase longevity. I thought getting old, tired, and sick was for other folks.

From an emotional point of view, I think when my myasthenia gravis really hit me the hardest was the period of several months beginning when Beth and I moved to our farm in early 1998 so I could focus on my health. This was the period when I started on the immunosuppressant therapy.

It was my idea to isolate myself. I imposed this self-isolation for three reasons: I felt I needed the solitude to rest my body. I felt so lousy much of the time that I didn't have much strength or energy for interacting effectively with others. And, quite candidly, I felt the steroids were going to trigger strange, hyperactive behavior in me; and I didn't want to embarrass myself in front of other people by acting out my personality changes around them.

It's one thing to make a decision you feel is the practical one to make. And that isolation decision was practical and in retrospect was a good investment in my getting back on a good track healthwise. However, it's another thing to live with a decision like that when it creates such a stark change in your lifestyle.

Quite frankly, it was gut-wrenching for me to deal with the isolation and boredom I experienced. I don't want to be tired; but I can tolerate it. However, I *surely* don't want to be bored. I cannot tolerate boredom. *It is extremely draining to me emotionally if I do not have a hill to climb.*

Also, I badly missed the friends and colleagues I was accustomed to seeing. In moving down to our rural, somewhat remote Twin Valley farm property, I did a thorough job in structuring this isolation. After we moved to the farm in 1998, I became so removed that I went for weeks or even months without seeing friends and colleagues I formerly had interacted with frequently. Beth and I weren't able to see our children and grandchildren as often. For me that isolation proved to be brutal! As active as I had been in so many areas, I recall feeling a degree of impotence and some helplessness. I missed being "in the arena."

From time to time during that period, Beth and I scheduled social occasions at the farm and invited people to visit. Sometimes that worked. Sometimes it didn't. We tried to schedule these social events when I was feeling decent. However, between the time we did the scheduling and when the event took place, my physical condition often deteriorated. I recall one incident when we had dear friends from Spartanburg, South Carolina, visiting us at the farm. I really was enjoying their visit. Then all of a sudden I came down with a brutal gastrointestinal virus and had to go to bed. I was too sick even to get out of bed and tell them goodbye when they left. I felt demoralized.

I am convinced this isolation issue deeply affects many chronic disease patients who encounter periods when they don't feel well enough to interact with others. I'm convinced there are many, many chronic disease patients out there who have days, weeks, or even months when they don't feel well enough to be around those they love; but at the same time they feel a gnawing, deep craving to enjoy this interaction.

Coming to Grips with Mortality

While I never came to grips with being isolated and bored—and I seriously doubt I ever will—after I became sick I did confront and come to grips with another very personal issue. I came to grips with my own mortality, with the prospect of my own death.

We all know we're going to die at some point. We face our mortality in different ways, at different times, depending on our views and what happens in our lives.

There is no doubt in my mind that I confronted my own mortality back in the late summer and early fall of 1995—that period just before my MG diagnosis, when I erroneously thought I had ALS, better known as Lou Gehrig's disease. At the time, I knew if the ALS diagnosis was accurate, it meant I would face imminent severe disability and death not far down the road. It was during that period in my life that I became at peace with dying. I have maintained that peace ever since. I can talk about it. I don't get emotional about it. I have incredible faith.

Concerned for the Family

Out of all the issues surrounding me about having MG, I think probably the most depressing thing was that I became such a weight on my wife and my family. I felt that as a major challenge.

When a chronic disease such as this hits someone, it severely impacts the entire family. My disease has impacted my beloved wife, Beth, our three children, our daughter-in-law and son-in-law, and our four grandchildren.

Of all my family members, the two who were spending the most time around me when MG initially came calling were Beth, who of course lived with me, and our son, Bill, who worked with me at MediSphere. It was hard on everyone in the family to watch me go downhill. However, it was right there staring Beth and Bill in the face all the time. Beth took on an increasing role as my primary support system and my primary caregiver. Where Bill was concerned, I felt particularly bad back in the 1995 and 1996 timeframe because my failing health placed him under even more pressure at MediSphere, at a time when the pressure already was off the chart.

I'll elaborate more about Beth later in this book, at the end of Chapter 7 on caregivers. For now, just suffice it to say that the strength of this woman is incredible, absolutely incredible. Without her, without her strength and her support to help me, I never would have made it back. It's as simple as that. Beth is my rock.

Bill did very touching things for me that I shall never forget. One thing he did back in my MediSphere days was to buy for me this big mattress-like contraption that you can blow up and use to take a nap on in your office. That thing is great! I started using it at MediSphere. Now, in my office at Twin Valley Farms, I still use it for naps. I'll tell the staff, "Don't interrupt me." And I plop down this convenient blow-up mattress Bill brought me and I lie down to get my all-important rest.

I remember an especially poignant conversation I had with Bill at the time I decided to become really candid with the family about my failing health. This was in 1995, at the time I went as far as to tell my family members that I thought I had ALS, or Lou Gehrig's disease. Bill and I were alone together on a plane trip. I was baring my soul about my health condition and my determination to go as far as I could go. I was telling him that I needed his support now more than ever. Compassionate, level-headed Bill just looked me in the eyes and said, "Dad, we're going to do whatever it takes. Whatever it takes, that's what we will do."

And then there have been the hundreds and hundreds of little daughter visits. The Rhonda and Ellen visits. The in-person visits. The phone visits. My daughters' questions, their concern, their love, their support. "How are you feeling? Do you need something? Could we just chat on the phone for a few minutes? When can we get together for dinner? Do you know how much I love you?" Rhonda and Ellen, just like their mother, there for me.

Our kids have married fine human beings. Son-in-law Tom is a strong and caring physician. Tom's father died two years after he and Rhonda married, and since then Tom and I have developed a relationship that truly is more like father and son. And daughter-in-law Lyn, well, Lyn knows me and has supported me from way back. She and I go back to the days when she was first my nurse and then our fertility nurse at Henderson & Walton Women's Center. To me, Tom and Lyn are like having another son and another daughter in the family.

I'm blessed. Before I came down with myasthenia gravis, I already knew I was blessed. But, since MG came along, I *really* know I am blessed.

Missing the Family

Ironically, it was at the same time myasthenia gravis entered my life that our family began to expand.

Beth and I had very much wanted to have grandchildren. We had been impatient to get them. When we started getting them, they came one after the other—four in three years, one boy and three girls. Grandson Matthew Thomas Powell was born to daughter Rhonda and husband Tom in 1994, and then granddaughter Lauren Elise was born to son Bill and wife Lyn in 1995. Rhonda and Tom had their second child, Caroline Elizabeth, in 1996. And Bill and Lyn had their second child, daughter Katherine Elizabeth, in 1997.

Beth and I are not the kind of grandparents who just want to dip in and out of their children's and grandchildren's lives periodically. We want to have frequent interaction. With our grandchildren as it has been with our children, we want to enjoy them, to help nurture them, to have impact in their lives. In fact, it bothered us at the time Matthew was born that Rhonda and Tom were living in Mississippi and we didn't get to see them as often as we liked. We were delighted when Rhonda and Tom decided to move to Alabama, and I greatly encouraged them to do so. After they moved, that meant that all our children and grandchildren were living in Birmingham, within a few miles of where Beth and I lived.

Considering how strongly I felt about family and the closeness of family, it was incredibly disturbing to me that myasthenia gravis entered my life the same year that the grandchildren began entering it. I can't begin to describe how frustrated I felt when my spells of illness and my diminished energy made it impossible to interact with my grandchildren to the degree that I wanted during the first years of their lives.

That early period with my MG, when I was out of touch so often, was hard on my family, too. After I imposed my self-isolation in early 1998 with the move to the farm, I didn't see the family as much.

We had been living at the farm for several months when I had a memorable conversation with our firstborn, daughter Rhonda, during one of her visits to the farm. As is typical with Rhonda, she was candid and to the point as she described a loss she was feeling. She said, "Papa, we moved back to Birmingham because you wanted us to. Now you've moved to the farm. We don't like it. We miss you. We want you and Mama B (Beth) back in Birmingham." I said, "Yes Ma'am."

Leveling Out

As I look back on the years 1999 and 2000 in my battle against myasthenia gravis, I think of them as "leveling-out years"—my bridge from the dark days to the light.

After many discussions between ourselves and also consulting other members of our family, in late 1998 Beth and I decided it was time to get back more in the mainstream of life. We gradually began spending more time in Birmingham, and in 1999 we bought and moved into a new home in Birmingham. My self-imposed isolation had officially ended. We started dividing our time between Twin Valley Farms and Birmingham.

I also began to travel a little—some personal, and some related to the beef business. The convenience of my return to some travel was helped along by the fact that I still could pilot my own plane. Following my diagnosis of myasthenia gravis, I had to wage a battle to retain my pilot's medical certificate. I was successful. In the course of that battle, I found there was little education about MG among those with authority over my medical certificate. At first after I was diagnosed with MG, my flight physical was conducted by a physician who had never seen a patient with MG. The physicians at the Federal Aviation Agency (FAA) understood that myasthenia gravis symptoms can be severe, but they did not understand how effectively treatments can control MG symptoms. After it was recommended that my medical certificate not be renewed, I was able to secure a medical opinion from a FAA doctor who did have experience in treating MG; and I succeeded in getting my medical certificate. I later found out that at the time my medical certificate was rejected I was the only private pilot in the United States with MG; now there are three. I feel that in being able to present my case successfully, this likely helped set a precedent for other MG patients who are well enough to pilot their planes.

Gradually, beginning in the latter part of 1999 and escalating in 2000 (when the full impact of the immunosuppressants began to kick in), I began to get my strength back. My MG symptoms were less, and I also was having fewer episodes of asthma and bronchitis. I became more involved in the business activities of Twin Valley Farms. I was attending bull sales. I was calling on some customers who were buying bulls from us. There came a point when I even felt strong enough to handle one of our big cattle sales. That was a milestone for me. The way I decided to approach it has become a mainstay with me in balancing activities with managing my MG. This approach simply is that I intersperse my activities with periods of rest for the MG. When I handled that first sale at the farm, over a day-and-a-half period I traveled back and forth several times between our sale barn and our farm home. I would make this short half-mile trip to our farm home and go to bed and rest, most of the time actually taking a nap, before I returned to the barn. That way, when I was back at the barn at work, I was strong and upbeat as I welcomed the crowd, hosted dinner meetings, and helped with the sale.

In April 2000, something wonderful happened, personally and pro-fessionally. I extended an invitation to our son, Bill, to take a full-time position working at Twin Valley Farms as the farm's business manager. At the time, Bill's heavy travel schedule in his position with MediSphere was leaving him little time at home with his wife, Lyn, and their two young daughters, Lauren and Katie. Too, Bill loved Twin Valley Farms. To my delight, Bill accepted; he joined Twin Valley on April 15, 2000. It was a good move for Bill and his family. It was good for Beth and me. Twin Valley is a LLC, a limited liability corporation. To make it a multi-generational business, you need a surviving member of the family to become actively involved. It was a comforting feeling to me to know that Bill would be my Twin Valley heir and successor.

As I began to feel stronger, I started spreading my wings further and further on both personal and business levels. Typical of my nature, I found it impossible to get involved in something to just a small extent.

I would get involved in a major way. Now that I was feeling stronger, it didn't seem that having myasthenia gravis had changed my tendency to get deeply involved. The only difference now was that I had to pace myself. Which I did. I began attending meetings of the Alabama chapter of the Myasthenia Gravis Foundation of America, Inc. (MGFA). One thing led to another, and for a time I served on the national board of that organization. On the business side, I got involved with a national business coalition called Future Beef. I helped this company's founders raise investment funds, and soon I found myself sitting as the chairman of Future Beef's board.

There are specific times I recall which served as uplifting turning points in my knowledge that I indeed was feeling better. One of those exhilarating occasions occurred in May of 2000. Looking back on it, I view it almost as a celebration that the full benefits of my longtime immunosuppressant therapy finally had taken hold. Beth and I were at the beach in Marco Island, Florida, for a Florida cattlemen's meeting. While there Beth and I were taking two walks a day on the beach. During one of those walks on the beach, all of a sudden it was just like a cloud lifted. I was stronger! I turned to Beth and said, "Darling, I feel differently. I don't know what it is. But I just feel different. I don't know if it will be permanent, or whether it's temporary or what. But I'm enjoying it!" Shortly thereafter, I returned to some weight-resistant exercising.

Only about four months after that, in the fall of 2000, I gradually started coming off the prednisone and Imuran®. I made the decision in the fall of 2000 that I wanted to come off both of them to the extent I could. My neurologist, Dr. Shin Oh, didn't agree with me, but I was committed to this. I had seen so many people on long-term immunosuppressant therapy who developed problems such as osteoporosis, obesity, and diabetes. So Dr. Oh worked with me in lowering the dosages of these medications. Now, these immunosuppressants are so powerful that you have to come off of them slowly. We gradually weaned me from the Imuran®; we went down from 150 milligrams to 50, then back up to 75, then slowly downward until I was off all Imuran®. With the prednisone, we came down gradually from my 60 milligrams a day to 5 milligrams a day. That had to be accomplished very slowly, and it was tough. I could feel the changes in my body as we went down on the dosage. There were times when I got to where I had to gut it out to achieve a lower dose. But slowly, slowly, slowly we did it. By the time I got down to 20 milligrams, we were going so slowly that I was lowering the dosage at a rate of one milligram less each week. It was worth it. When I got down to my 5 milligrams-a-day maintenance dosage of prednisone, I felt like someone I used to know—the old Ron Henderson.

All in all, beginning in 2001, I was losing the feeling that this disease called MG was keeping me down; and instead I was beginning to feel that I was getting on top of the disease.

4

Traveling a Brighter Road

If someone were to ask me to identify one key message I want to impress upon every reader of this book, I wouldn't have to ponder my answer. *That key message is this: What's most important in charting your future is not so much what happens in your life; what's most important is what you do with what happens in your life.*

I have believed that axiom to be true since even before I reached adulthood. In various ways, my mother and father both stressed that philosophy. Never had I realized just *how* true it was until I had to learn to live with a chronic disease—in my case, myasthenia gravis.

For many reasons, some of which I'll mention in this chapter, I can tell you that my life today is less limited than it was prior to my first MG symptoms eight years ago. As I write this in the year 2002, I can truthfully tell you that my life is fuller than it has ever been in my 65 years. I'm stronger emotionally and spiritually; I'm incredibly active; and, because I'm taking care of myself and responding well to treatment, I'm doing well physically.

In short, life is good. I feel as though I have a new lease on life.

A Need to Reach Out to Others

In the early days of my battle against myasthenia gravis, one of the things that bothered me most was not being able to muster the strength and stamina I needed to reach out to help others. On the contrary, others were having to reach out to help me.

Most of us feel better about ourselves when we get our minds off our own needs and reach out to help someone else. However, I'll have to admit that during the early period of dealing with MG there were all too many days when I was focused very inwardly. I was focused on what I could do to get Ron Henderson back on the road to a healthier life.

For me this self-absorption was an uncomfortable feeling in a couple of ways. For one thing, I had experienced so little illness in my life that I didn't have much practice with being sick and having to concentrate on getting better. The one notable exception was my being involved in a 1974 car accident. Although I sustained severe injuries in that accident and was hospitalized for weeks, that road to recovery was not nearly as long as the worst months of my MG. Too, unlike with a chronic disease, there was some kind of end in sight to my recovery period following the accident. With MG, I had to become accustomed to ongoing, never-ending management of the disease.

Another reason I felt uncomfortable with focusing so much on myself after I got MG was that it felt strange to be the one who was in need, rather than the one who was meeting other people's needs. In my longtime role as a physician, it had been my job and mission for decades to focus on the needs of the many people who came to me with their health problems. I had little experience with having to turn to others for help with my own health challenges.

Thus, in early 2001 it was a rewarding experience for me to again be able to reach out in a major way to help someone else in need.

That someone else was my mother-in-law, Elizabeth Summerville.

The Gift of Elizabeth

It was January 18, 2001, when Beth's mother, Elizabeth, suffered a massive coronary. She was 89 years old. The attack was physically devastating, claiming 80 percent of her cardiac function and leaving her with a prognosis of death within a short period of time.

Elizabeth was treated in the hospital for several weeks. Then Beth and I had her transferred to our home at Twin Valley Farms to spend the final days of her life. Beth and I joined forces with a hospice program and Elizabeth's physician, Dr. Walker Brown, in taking care of Elizabeth at our farm home. She died just shy of a month later, on March 10.

That experience was incredibly special—I would venture to say even sacred—for both Beth and me. Beth ministered to Elizabeth's basic needs, I coordinated the overall management of Elizabeth's healthcare, and we both showered Elizabeth with large dosages of our love and attention.

Beth and I both believe so strongly in being able to die with dignity. Over the years, the subject of death with dignity has been featured in articles I have written and many speeches I have delivered. Elizabeth indeed did die with dignity. As she interacted with us in her own way during her final days, Elizabeth obviously was at peace and very aware she was in loving surroundings.

It was around 2 a.m. when I received the telephone call from Beth that Elizabeth had suffered the attack. I was in Orlando, Florida, on business. And I was trying to fight off one of those bouts with bronchitis and asthma—bouts that by that time were at least becoming less frequent and less severe. I got on the telephone to locate the physician I wanted to care for Elizabeth, and I arrived back home the next day.

When I saw for myself the toll this attack had taken on Elizabeth, it was a little difficult for me to comprehend that this was actually real, that this really had happened to her. Many of us have loved ones in our family who just seem invincible. Well, Elizabeth was that kind of person. She had always been so active, so full of herself. Elizabeth was very social and knew virtually everyone in her hometown of Prattville. She was proud and well groomed, and she wore those high heels with the grace of a woman half her age. Even as Elizabeth advanced into her late 80s, there were days when super-active Beth had trouble keeping up with her mother.

Elizabeth was unique and so spirited that she really didn't have to do anything in order for her presence to transform even the most structured event into something unusual. Thus, I think it was somewhat in keeping with her personality that even her trip to the hospital the night of her attack did not turn out to be ordinary. The ambulance was involved in a wreck, and Elizabeth had to be transferred to another ambulance just to make it to the hospital.

While Elizabeth was in the hospital, she was on a ventilator for a short time. When she came off, due to some cause we can't identify for sure, she was paralyzed from the neck down. But even in that condition, Elizabeth managed to communicate with Beth and me during the last weeks of her life. She couldn't talk, but she surely could mouth words and we could tell what those words were. Her face was partially paralyzed, but even with that she managed to be expressive.

I look back on that experience as being *the gift of Elizabeth*. It was a situation of mutual giving. No matter how much Beth and I did for Elizabeth, we felt that she was giving back even more to us.

Something else came out of that experience, too. Taking care of Elizabeth got my clinical juices to flowing. I started thinking about returning on a part-time basis to the practice of medicine. Today I still view that as an option.

Filling Up that Schedule

All my life I had been busy. I thrived on having my plate run over with activities, on always having a project in the wings. In the year 2000, as soon as I sighted real light in the tunnel with getting my MG under control, I got busier and busier—in both business and volunteer roles. I think one good thing fed another; feeling better got me more involved, and being more involved made me feel better.

As general manager of Twin Valley Farms, I was glowing with pride as that beef-farming operation became more and more successful. I found myself at many beef sales, hosting beef-related events at the farm, and enjoying my interaction with our staff and customers.

Still serving as a board member of MediSphere, I was continuing to hold high hopes for this company I had founded a decade ago. The company had some new initiatives about which I was enthused.

As a leader in Future Beef, I became embroiled in a business saga of highs and lows. After showing phenomenal promise in 1999 and 2000, Future Beef encountered challenges in late 2001 with a troubled international beef market and a recession. Then, along with many other business ventures in this nation, Future Beef was dealt a huge blow by the terrorist attacks of September 11, 2001. In the aftermath of the attacks, Future

Beef felt the harsh sting of severe declines in lucrative markets such as high-end dining. Through this rough ride, I had to call upon some of those stress-management tools I had learned to practice in recent years. I made it a point to practice stress management, and it worked.

As members of both the communities of Birmingham, Alabama, and Prattville, Alabama, Beth and I feel a strong need to pay our civic rent. As I began feeling better, we stepped up both our church and civic activities. In Prattville, we became avid supporters of and contributors to the local YMCA. In Birmingham, we became more active in our church, Mountain Brook Baptist. And, also in Birmingham, I enjoyed my service as a board member of the St. Vincent's Hospital Foundation, at the hospital where I had practiced for many years.

It was important to me to leave time to do some volunteer work related to myasthenia gravis. I became vice president and then president of the Alabama Chapter of the Myasthenia Gravis Foundation of America, Inc. Beth and I hosted a fundraiser for that organization at Twin Valley Farms in October 2001. And in early 2002 I got busy setting up a new foundation to be dedicated to myasthenia gravis research. The goal with that new foundation is that knowledge can be uncovered about MG that will combat not only MG but also other autoimmune diseases as well. As I placed myself in the role of MG educator and fundraiser, it became necessary for me to go public with the fact I have MG. Since my mother and Beth's mother now were deceased, and since a major reason for keeping my MG secret had been for them not to know, I felt free to do interviews with the media that included my own MG story. I still was not comfortable with it, but I felt I was doing it for a good cause.

Taking Care of My Health

The healthy lifestyle regimen I now use has as its cornerstone the same four basic tenets that I used for my health-maintenance regimen prior to getting MG. I've continued that old regimen, and I have added to it the new MG regimen.

These are the four tenets of the old basic healthy-living regimen that I practiced even prior to MG and which I continue to practice today:

- **Number one, I don't smoke.** I have never smoked, and I never will.
- **Number two, I watch my weight.** I stay between 165 and 170 pounds.
- **Number three, I eat a balanced diet.** I eat eight helpings of fresh fruits and vegetables daily, try to drink two gallons of water a day, and don't eat pasta, rice, or potatoes. If I want a dessert, I eat yogurt or occasionally sorbet. To keep my weight under control, I don't eat anything within three hours of going to bed.
- **Number four, I exercise daily.** After I awaken, have my period of meditation, and take my morning medicines, I dress for exercise. I usually work out from 7 a.m. until 8 a.m. Also every day I enjoy some kind of aerobic activity—perhaps an hour walk, maybe a 30-minute jog.

I sincerely feel that my adherence over the years to those basic four healthy lifestyle tenets has helped prevent my MG condition from being worse than it has been. I think I have been aided in working my way back from MG by the positives of being in good physical condition, having never smoked, exercising routinely, and eating healthily. Too, I think I likely have been spared a critical MG breathing crisis because of being in good physical condition. I know now that I have needed all the edge I could get. Even with being in good overall physical shape, I came awfully close to suffering a MG breathing crisis; it just never became full-blown.

In addition to my four basic healthy lifestyle habits, I have added to my regimen four new MG-related disciplines:

- **I take my medicines faithfully.** Currently I'm taking the following: prednisone to keep my immune system in check (but only 5 milligrams every other day!), Mestinon® for muscle weakness, Robinal® to control the Mestinon®-related side effect of diarrhea, Klonopin® to control muscle twitching, Singulair® for asthma, Claritin® to suppress allergies that might aggravate asthma, and, a new drug about which I'm very excited for both men and women, Fosamax® to prevent osteoporosis.
- **I am careful not to expose myself to infections.** Since my immune

system is depressed, I am subject to infections. I am vigilant about taking my flu shot, and I have had my pneumonia shot. After shaking hands with anyone, I wash my hands. And I watch out for people with upper respiratory infections and try to stay away from them.

- **I cooperate and interact with my physicians to manage my healthcare.** Since coming down with MG, I've learned the importance of becoming the quarterback of my own treatment team. I keep up to date about what's going on with MG treatments, I'm knowledgeable, and I ask questions and express opinions.
- **No doubt the most difficult of the new tenets for me to live by has been making sure I get rest.** If I don't have a rest period during one day, the next day I'm likely to require twice as much rest. Too, I've had to learn to balance my appointments and activities in a way that allows me to delay or even cancel an appointment when I need to. Since I had never allowed myself that flexibility prior to MG, exercising those rescheduling options from time to time really bothered me at first. But I have learned to do it. Myasthenia gravis demands that you get rest and that you pace yourself, so I've learned to lie down for rest periods during the day and to structure my schedule carefully.

Strengthened by My Parents

From the time I was born, my parents instilled in me an upbringing of strength, discipline, and positive thinking that has served me well during my battle against myasthenia gravis.

I was reared on a modest farm in the central Alabama county of Autauga. Since I was born in 1937, my upbringing was influenced by the economic hardships in the wake of the Great Depression and by the scarcity and rationing of the World War II years. While our parents' hard work ensured that we had food to eat and clothes to wear, my two younger brothers and I were reared in an environment where money was scarce and hard farm work was plentiful. That meant not only hard work for the adults, but for us boys as well.

Mental toughness was demonstrated on a daily basis by both my mother and my father, as well as by my maternal grandmother, who lived right across the road from us. I was never exposed to my parents demonstrating self-pity, and I was never allowed to feel sorry for myself. I was always told I was blessed.

It was an environment in which there was no hill too big to climb. Whatever tasks you had to do on a given day, you did them. There were no questions about it. When severe economic challenges came—and they came often—those challenges were faced and dealt with. When cataclysmic life events occurred in the family—like my grandmother getting very sick or my dad being in an automobile wreck—the family faced those thngs and went on. I was taught that when good things happen you enjoy them, and when bad things happen you deal with them.

As an example, I remember a situation that occurred when I was a youngster. I was just five years old when I sustained a severe cut on my foot that became infected and I contracted septicemia, or "blood poisoning" as we called it then. Those were the days prior to penicillin, and septicemia in that day and time often was fatal, particularly in children. My situation was serious enough that the doctor was coming t our house every day to tend to me. However, aside from my being able to read grave concern on my mother's face, I received no indication from anyone in the family that I was n jeopardy. It was just understood that I was going to survive and do all right.

As I grew into adulthood and better understood the backgrounds of my parents, I had more insights into the challenges they had encountered which had been factors in molding their own strength and discipline. Dad and Mother complemented one another in their styles and teachings as parents. Dad was so focused and driven to work hard, and Mother voiced a consistent message about the need to get an education. I greatly benefited from both parents.

My dad, William Earl Henderson, was an exceptionally intelligent man who did not have the opportunity for higher education because of the harsh economic limitations of the times. It was the year 1929—the year of the "official" birth of the Great Depression—when Dad graduated magna cum laude from Sidney Lanier High School in Alabama's capital city of Montgomery. Although Dad could have attended college his first year for a total of $300, the shortage of money prevented him from doing so.

Many times as a young man, Dad faced grim money challenges. It was toward the end of my dad's life, during a period when he and I were especially close, when Dad confided in me just how hard he had to scrape to make ends meet at various times in his life. At one point, there had been a period when he worked as a migrant farm worker in Oklahoma and the Texas Panhandle.

My dad was a hard-working farmer by day and a voracious reader at night. He was a driven, confident man. Dad taught me about hard work, he taught me to learn through the written word, and, through his example, he taught me about self-confidence. On the hard work side, Dad without a doubt had the most brutal work ethic of anybody I've ever worked with at any time in my life. He didn't just *teach* me to work hard; he *expected* me to work hard. On the learning side, Dad encouraged me to do a lot of things that a rural Alabama boy in that period typically would not have been doing. For example, as a teenager I read *The Power of Positive Thinking* by Dr. Norman Vincent Peale. On the positive-thinking, self-confidence side, Dad encouraged me to enter a countywide "pig-chain contest" that attracted some 350 to 400 contestants. I became one of six winners. As a prize I won my own pig, and as a bonus I gained in self-confidence.

It took me awhile to realize that Dad also had been a masterful psychologist during my growing-up years. It never was my dad's style to compliment me. But he did something that in the long run might well have served me better. He *showed* his high opinion of me by treating me as his peer. His doing that proved to be one of the great molders of my life.

My mother, Sara Dillard Henderson, started encountering major struggles at the tender age of 12 when her mother died. Her father married two more times; the circumstances that unfolded only brought more sadness to my mother during her teenage years. For all practical purposes, Mother was orphaned from age 12.

Instead of defeating her, the unhappy life Mother lived as a teenager galvanized her strength and molded her into an exceptionally determined and proud adult. An attractive, well-groomed, high-energy woman with an incredibly positive spirit, Mother became extremely ambitious. Her ambition was especially directed toward furthering the lives of three individuals, three boys to whom she affectionately referred as "My Three Sons"—my younger brothers, Jerry and Tommy, and me.

From the time I can remember, Mother always planned for her sons to go to college. And we all went. I can recall her telling me often, "Now, Ronnie, I want you to be a doctor, lawyer, or a minister." To all three of her sons, she was constantly teaching personal growth, positive attitude, and a can-do attitude. We listened. It was easy to listen to Mother about those things, because she practiced what she preached.

My brothers and I were not the only ones who benefited from Mother's encouragement. Mother touched so many people in the Alabama town of Prattville, which was located a few miles from our farm and thus was our "hometown." She interacted with a lot of people in her work, because she had a job in which she dealt with the public. To make it possible for the family to have more and also to give what little economic boost she could toward her sons' college education, Mother went to work as a cashier in a Prattville supermarket and rapidly became head cashier. On a daily basis, as she checked out groceries for the townspeople, Mother touched many with her kindness and her upbeat attitude. At her funeral, it was so special to me that one person after another came up to me and told his or her own story about having been so positively impacted by my mother.

Inspired by My Brothers

Just as I feel I was strengthened by the upbringing I received from my parents, I know I have been inspired by the examples my younger brothers have set for me. The brother closest in age to me is Gerald Eugene Henderson, better known as Jerry. He's three years my junior. The youngest in the family, nine years younger than I, is Thomas Elbert Henderson, better known as Tommy.

My brothers have lived highly productive, successful, and enjoyable lives despite the fact that both have waged a lifelong battle against the severe blood disease known as hemophilia. Jerry and Tommy were born with classical hemophilia, an inherited blood-clotting defect that affects only males. Individuals suffering from hemophilia have a shortage of the protein necessary to make the blood clot, a defect that places them at risk for hemorrhaging.

Through the years, Jerry and Tommy have undergone multiple rounds of therapy, including numerous treatments with blood products. As a side effect to undergoing blood transfusions, both have developed hepatitis C. They have suffered many episodes of bleeding profusely—bleeding associated with surgeries and injuries, and also even with routine dental extractions and simple lacerations. Too, they have suffered repeated gastro-intestinal bleedings and bleeding into the joints. Today Jerry and Tommy still experience bleeding episodes. Because they are at such high-risk for hemorrhaging due to their hemophilia, neither is a candidate for a liver transplant, which is the most effective treatment for hepatitis C. Thus, as is the case with me and my chronic disease, Jerry and Tommy can only hope that cures will be found for both of the chronic diseases they face.

Despite the numerous obstacles my two brothers have confronted, extending from childhood into adulthood, they have gone forward with their lives. Neither has ever had a "woe is me" attitude. Jerry and Tommy have done what they have had to do. They have been responsible. They have been busy being productive. They have been busy enjoying life. That's what they continue to do today.

In high school, Jerry and Tommy played basketball and baseball and were class leaders. In college, Jerry earned a business degree; and Tommy earned a degree in electrical engineering. In their careers, Jerry and Tommy have excelled and have continued to show leadership ability.

Now retired, Jerry began his career with Standard Oil of Kentucky and later joined Chevron International. In the latter years of his career, Jerry was a high-level Chevron International executive based in San Francisco.

Tommy still is in the prime of his successful longtime career with International Paper.

In both my brothers I see a uniqueness of positive spirit. Although they have this severe genetic-linked disease, they just accept it as an ongoing challenge that requires and receives special management. They manage it, and go on. Each day, they live with the disease as an accepted part of their day. In their thoughts and actions, they don't dwell on hemophilia. They live normal lives.

During the time I secluded myself on my farm in Prattville with the goal of dealing with my MG and getting better physically, Jerry and Tommy served as a real inspiration to me. During my most severe "valley times" during that period, I would think of the examples that had been set by Jerry and Tommy; and that inspired me to go forward.

During that difficult period, Jerry and Tommy came to the farm to visit with Beth and me. While we visited with one another, we talked about a lot of things; but we talked very little about my MG. I found myself settling in to where Jerry and Tommy had been for so long. I was beginning to accept my chronic disease as a part of my life, and going forward with a life that was becoming more and more normal in spite of my disease. Nowadays when I talk by phone with my brothers, or when we visit in person, we spend very little time talking about myasthenia gravis, hemophilia, and hepatitis C. In the back of our minds, all three of us know we are dealing with chronic disease. *We also know we are excited to be able to live productively in spite of our chronic diseases.* When we have our brotherly conversations, we are all too happy to talk about the interesting, exciting things we are doing with our lives.

That All-Important Positive Attitude

Most mornings when I awaken I feel really good, ready to go. On some other days, however, I don't feel that energetic. That's the basic nature of myasthenia gravis; it's a cyclic disease, characterized by ups and downs. You might feel great one morning, and the next day it could be hard to get out of bed. The unpredictability of MG is just something that you have to learn to live with.

But, all in all, I'm doing well and my overall energy level continues to be on the rise. The thing that I make sure is constant, no matter if

I'm feeling on top of the world or a little energy-deprived, is that I keep my attitude positive. I've been successful in doing that.

I think having a positive attitude is all-important in dealing with any chronic disease. In fact, I think having a negative attitude toward a chronic disease is almost analogous to having a death wish. You just have to persist, to keep going forward. To have a negative attitude injures your immune system, and this obviously is detrimental to keeping you on a healthy track. I think two great therapies when you have a chronic disease are laughter and learning. Back when I was so sick, I would listen to tapes that made me laugh. As for learning, when you have a chronic disease you need to stretch your mind—to read and learn. Right now I'm trying to learn more about the computer.

Having MG has taught me a lot. For one thing, it has reaffirmed my mentality about not looking at the problem, but looking for a solution. For me, I think the three things most responsible for my finding some solutions to getting back on a road to a healthier life have been my positive attitude, my persistence in working with my doctors to look for a combination of treatment modalities, and the wonderful, loving support I've received from family and friends.

I have been blessed in terms of support. I have indeed been overwhelmed by the support of my family and my friends. And let me tell you, those four grandchildren of mine have been magical potions of therapy and enjoyment! One of the joys of my feeling better is that I'm having such a great time with them. When I look at my precious grandchildren, I think of my new goal—to see my great-grandchildren.

Facing Reality—and *Still* Staying Positive

One thing that keeps my positive attitude intact is confronting the reality that my disease is chronic, that I can't just snap my fingers or take a magic pill and make MG go away. That way, I'm not continually frustrated; I'm grounded and I go on and live my life and manage my MG.

I think any person who has a chronic, incurable disease has to come to grips with that—whether you're dealing with MG, multiple sclerosis, diabetes, rheumatoid arthritis, whatever. That's really where you have to get with a chronic disease. The disease sticks with you, so you have to learn to ride with it.

When you're dealing with a chronic disease, it's very different from an acute illness, injury, or intervention brought on by something like a bad case of flu, a car accident, or a surgical procedure. Dealing with a chronic disease means that you have to learn to be at home with the disease. Oh, you can hold out hope for a cure or a miracle drug or a re-mission. You can even work in some way to try to make these wonderful things happen. And you should never stop looking for solutions. But, at the same time, you have to take a realistic approach to your disease. You must view your chronic disease as something you must live with and manage—as though, under the best scenario, your chronic disease is a semi-permanent part of your life.

After I was diagnosed with myasthenia gravis, I did a lot of reading about my disease. I would urge anyone with a chronic disease to do the same thing. It became natural to me that I began to view the handling of my myasthenia gravis like I had handled any other challenge in my life. I knew that with myasthenia gravis, my challenge was to manage the disease. You either manage the disease or it manages you. *I'm viewing the management of my chronic disease as just another hill to climb.*

PART TWO

MESSAGES FOR KEY AUDIENCES: PATIENTS, PHYSICIANS, CAREGIVERS, AND COMMUNITIES

5

Patients, Take Charge!

Once you have been diagnosed with a chronic disease, the first thing you should do is make up your mind to take charge of the management of your disease. You must do what I refer to as "take ownership" of your disease.

If you think management of your disease is primarily the responsibility of your doctor or doctors, you're wrong. You hire your doctors to be your guides and facilitators in managing your disease, and you consult with your doctors periodically. However, you live with your chronic disease all the time, and you must be the one to manage it. From my dual points of view as a physician and a chronic disease patient, there's no doubt in my mind that managing chronic disease *must* become the responsibility of the patient who has that disease, if the patient has the capability.

In the case of a patient who is so compromised physically, emotionally, and/or mentally that he or she can't take charge, it's very important for a family member, friend, or designated caretaker to assume this take-charge responsibility on behalf of the patient.

If neither the patient nor the patient's advocate succeeds in taking charge and assuming disease ownership, then the patient is at risk of becoming a pawn of the healthcare system. By that I mean that the patient might have to take potluck with whatever the healthcare system happens to do or not do for him. Consequently, the patient is at risk for lack of care, inappropriate care, and poorly managed care.

What do I mean by taking ownership of your disease? The following are my 12 basic rules in assuming ownership and taking charge of managing your chronic disease.

RULE NUMBER 1: Educate yourself about your disease. Knowledge is power. Make it your goal to become so knowledgeable about your disease that you know more about it than your doctor. Learn about the treatments for the disease and the pros and cons of having those treatments. Educate yourself about the medications that typically are used and what side effects are involved. Know about new treatments that are on the horizon. Learn about research that's being conducted on your disease. To become informed, seek out creditable information from health-related organizations and governmental health agencies. For a start, take these steps: Visit your library, go to appropriate websites, procure pamphlets and fact sheets, and interview your physicians and other experts in the field. Also, if it matches your needs, join and attend informational meetings sponsored by a support group that represents your disease.

RULE NUMBER 2: Practice the four basic tenets of a "healthy living" lifestyle. I've practiced these healthy lifestyle habits for decades. They have paid off for me and continue to pay off. These four healthy living tenets can improve your chances of living a productive life despite your chronic disease. Also, they can help prevent your developing other chronic health problems. While you can't change the genetic package your mother and father gave you that might put you at risk for this health problem or that one, you can reduce those risks via these positive daily habits. If you were not already practicing these four tenets prior to being diagnosed with a chronic disease, it's essential that you start doing so. If you were practicing them, you must continue. As you live this healthy lifestyle, be aware that you are among a disciplined minority. Studies show that only three percent of our American population adheres to these four principles. They are: *First of all, do not smoke.* Smoking is a brutal thing to do to your body. *Secondly, maintain a normal body weight.* Your doctor and standard health insurance charts can tell you how much you should weigh according to your height, body build, gender, and age. *Thirdly, eat a balanced diet.* I use a diet that includes eating at least eight daily servings of fresh fruits and vegetables, and drinking *lots* of water. You will have to match the makeup of your balanced diet to the demands of whatever chronic disease you might have. For example, you will have special diet indications if you have diabetes. *And fourth and last, practice a daily, disciplined regimen of physical exercise.* For the general population, this means at least two hours of exercise a week, including aerobic exercise. But here again, you must tailor your exercise program to your own individual capabilities. I recommend that you consult an expert to help you plan your exercise regimen. I can't tell you how strongly I believe in the benefits of physical exercise—as a tool for controlling weight, maintaining overall body strength and healthy bones, strengthening your immune system, improving your mental outlook, and managing stress.

RULE NUMBER 3: Practice mental exercise. Exercise your mind. Continue to study and learn. Now that you have a chronic disease, it's more important than ever that you stay as sharp as possible and on top of things. Just as physical exercise is important, so is mental exercise. If you don't use your brain, your brainpower will diminish and your thinking and focus will become sluggish. One way you can stretch your mind is to conduct research on your disease, and pack your brain with facts about your disease. In addition to that, I strongly recommend you find something new you want to learn that has nothing to do with your disease. Find a new hobby, a new cause, or a new interest. This could be energizing, fun, and productive. Perhaps consider taking some community school classes or even a college or trade school course.

RULE NUMBER 4: Balance rest with activity. It's important that a chronic disease patient get a sufficient amount of rest. Now that you know you must manage a chronic disease, you might need to adjust your schedule to accommodate naps and/or an increased number of regular sleeping hours. At the same time, it's important that you not rest too much. You must remain active; you must continue to be involved in life and with people as much as possible. Don't sleep your life away. Since I have been diagnosed with myasthenia gravis, I have made sure I have enough rest to minister to my MG and also to give me the fuel I need for my active life. I have added rest periods to my schedule, including naps either in my office or at home. Otherwise, I still adhere mostly to the regular sleeping pattern I practiced even back in my busiest days as a physician. Usually I'm in bed by 9 p.m. and asleep by 10. Each morning I awaken and get up without the aid of an alarm clock. I'm an early riser, starting my day around 4:30 to 5 a.m. My early-morning quiet time is important to me. Immediately after I arise—even before I take my morning medicines, exercise, and have breakfast—I enjoy a period of quiet time. During that period, I meditate, pray, write, prepare my "to do" list for the day, and enjoy some favorite television news and talk-show programs. I find that period first thing in the morning is a great investment in the serenity and organization with which I approach my day. Once I've finished my early-morning routine of quiet time, medicines, exercise, and breakfast, I embark on an active day interrupted only by an afternoon nap to refuel.

RULE NUMBER 5: Interact productively with your doctor or doctors as an active partner in the management of your chronic disease. Keep in mind *you* are the one who ultimately is in charge. *One thing you must do in order to interact productively with your doctor is to ask the doctor questions that are important to you, and express yourself if you have doubts about, or a lack of understanding of, what the doctor is doing.* I think oftentimes it's difficult for a layperson to bring himself to ask hard questions of the doctor. However, if the questions are on your mind, you must ask them. Again, informing yourself about your disease is all-important here—so you'll have the information you need to make sure you're asking all the questions you need to ask. Some of your questions to your doctor might be: "Why are you putting me on this medicine? Why are you approaching my chronic disease with these particular treatments? What research do you have to back up this treatment approach? Has this approach worked in other patients?" *Another thing you must do to interact productively with your doctor is to follow the doctor's advice about treatments he prescribes, once the two of you have agreed these treatments are appropriate for you.* Over the years in my role as a physician, I would tell my patients, "You come in here and tell me what's wrong with you, and then I'll try to tell you what

I think will help you. However, I'm not effective if you're not going to follow what I say." *The last bit of advice I would give you in dealing with your doctor is to be honest with him.* If you're feeling bad, tell him you're feeling bad; and describe clearly how you feel. If you haven't taken the medicines your doctor has prescribed, tell him that. I personally know what it's like not to be totally honest with your doctor. I wasn't honest with mine prior to being diagnosed with myasthenia gravis. The reason was that I didn't want to admit to myself how bad I was feeling—I was in denial—so I didn't admit it to my doctor. Instead, I diagnosed myself, and I made a mistake with the self-diagnosis. I think there is an attitude among some people, especially males, which makes them tend to not admit they're sick. Call them "type A personalities," call them "alpha male personalities," whatever handle you want to put on it. It's people who are self-contained to the point of arrogance, even stupidity, in their approach to health and longevity. This type of personality on the part of the patient can create a barrier to being properly diagnosed and treated.

RULE NUMBER 6: Maintain a positive attitude. This is a key theme I'm trying to hammer home again and again in this book. As a chronic disease patient, it's imperative that you have a positive attitude. There are millions of people living productive lives in spite of the fact they suffer from chronic disease. We all have our challenges in life. I've stated the following previously in this book, and I believe it so strongly I'll state it again: What's most important in charting your future is not so much what happens in your life; what's most important is what you do with what happens in your life. You *can* turn lemons into lemonade. Just because you have a chronic health problem, you can't look at it as "woe is me." There are phenomenal examples out there of patients with chronic health problems who have taken the high road—including patients with huge challenges. Obviously actor Christopher Reeve is incredibly qualified to serve as one of our role models. Famous for portraying the fictitious "Superman," Chris became a real-life superman to us all after he became a quadriplegic. He turned his disaster into a positive by raising money aimed at finding a cure for many who have suffered spinal injuries. To anyone who has a chronic health problem, I say it's in your own interest to stay positive. I know that sometimes it's awfully difficult for a chronic disease patient not to get depressed, that it's very difficult to refrain from looking at the glass as half-empty. However, for you, for your family, for the good of your immune system as you strive to live a productive life, it's essential you see that glass as half-full. You must focus on staying spiritually and emotionally grounded, on looking forward and not backward, on looking outward and not inward.

RULE NUMBER 7: **Minimize and manage the stress in your life.** I am not recommending here that you endeavor to eliminate all stress from your life. We all have stress in our lives. What I'm saying is that to the degree you can, avoid getting yourself into extremely stressful situations. I recommend that you find effective ways to manage whatever stress you do encounter. This might mean reading some books on stress management or taking a course in stress management. I think there are trends in today's society that are increasing the stress to which we're exposed. Our communities are going away; at least, the closeknit, caring nature of our communities sadly is becoming less prevalent. There's less and less matrix in our communities, and there's less structure in our lives. Too, people are living longer and society is becoming more complicated. There's a particular reason that you as a chronic disease patient must take control of stress rather than letting it control you. That reason is protecting your immune system. In order for you to combat your chronic disease and to keep your overall body as strong as possible, you must pamper your immune system. I strongly believe the immune system is wired so that it does not work well at all if you have harmful stress. In patients with autoimmune diseases such as myasthenia gravis, I think stress probably often plays a big part in injuring the immune system. In my daily life now since I've been diagnosed with myasthenia gravis, I try to communicate effectively and efficiently without losing my temper; and I discipline myself not to worry. I even try not to get in a rush.

RULE NUMBER 8: **Don't focus on your chronological age.** Instead, try to enhance your age biologically by taking care of your health and staying active. Practice the four tenets of healthy living that I outlined in Rule Number 2, and also partner with your doctors in managing your chronic disease. Beyond that, enjoy your family and friends, get involved in activities, and energize your life by launching new projects. Instead of focusing on how old you are, focus on doing something new that could be exciting and energizing. That something new could be a project such as renovating your home or having an addition built on, learning how to play golf or tennis, becoming proficient with the computer, or researching and writing your family's genealogy. All my life I've thrived on new projects; I still do. On the general subject of becoming depressed about one's chronological age, I venture to say that in general men are more likely to do that than are women. That's ironic, considering how much women are teased about vanity, trying to roll back the years, and in some cases being reluctant to tell their age. However, having been a physician to thousands of women over the years, I really do think women have a stronger tendency to age productively than do men. It's especially common for men who live well beyond retirement age to become reclusive, withdraw from life, stop growing, and often to start dying emotionally and spiritually years before the final words are said at their funerals. I wish many older, depressed men could meet a Nebraska man who is a friend of mine. He is 85 years old, he continues to look forward, and he has just bought a new ranch and built a new home! In closing on this Rule Number 8, I want to emphasize that when I say you shouldn't focus on your chronological age, that doesn't mean that you deny your age. I'm proud to tell anyone I'm 65. What I'm saying is that you should view your age as a positive and keep going forward.

RULE NUMBER 9: Don't isolate yourself. As a patient suffering from a chronic disease, you must make an extra effort to resist becoming isolated and instead to arrange interaction with other people. By interacting with other people, you can be stimulated by conversation and laughter, stay informed on what's going on around you, and be nurtured by the companionship of others. As one suffering from a chronic disease, you also can help others. Living with a chronic disease has given you a special understanding of what it's like to face challenges. If you so choose, you likely can be effective in reaching out to help others who are isolated. That can be a win-win situation. You can help the other person and also get your mind off your own problems. I've always been a people person, always had interaction with many groups of people on a daily basis. Since I have had myasthenia gravis, I've had reason to reflect on the high value of interaction with people. I treasure that interaction. Beth and I make it a point to schedule time with our family and friends. If I don't call all three of my children every day, they call me. When I hear of a loved one who needs an encouraging word, I pick up the phone or pay a visit. In 1998, I learned from personal experience how brutal isolation can be. I learned that lesson during a period that year when I imposed a period of isolation upon myself in order to rest and get back on track healthwise. There could come a time when you, too, need a short period of isolation. My advice to you is to keep any period of isolation as short as possible. I really do believe that one of the most damaging things with chronic disease is the isolation that often accompanies it. Many times an individual will isolate himself or herself not only because of not feeling well but also because of being depressed. We see that particularly in an older person who has lost a spouse. We see it in individuals who do not have a core support group of family and friends in the community where they live. Isolation can be insidious. Sometimes without even realizing it a person becomes more and more reclusive. This can lead to a pattern that is sad, damaging, and potentially deadly—one in which a person can become reclusive to the point that he or she does not get adequate nutrition, doesn't get seen by a doctor on a regular basis, and doesn't receive medicines on time. It can be a vicious cycle that just gets worse and worse. On the education side, there are limited ways we can reach reclusive chronically ill patients as long as they are sick and/or depressed. We can try to help them by giving them reading materials, but often they won't read them. Human contact—living, breathing, personal contact from caring people—holds the strongest chance of helping these people. Often that human contact ends up coming from somebody who is not sick—a spouse, daughter, son, relative, friend, or even a caring outsider. Also, I emphasize again that patients who are coping successfully with their own chronic health problems, and who are active and involved in life, often can be effective in reaching out to help other chronically ill patients who have fallen victim to isolation. If you know someone who is isolated and you think you can help that person, do it. *You will be handsomely rewarded.*

RULE NUMBER 10: Don't stop looking for solutions to the problems you face with your chronic disease. Of all 12 of these rules, none is stronger than this. Do not stop investigating what's out there for you—what's out there in the form of treatments and approaches to managing your chronic disease. Don't become complacent with having your chronic disease managed the same old way indefinitely. The more severe and the more chronic your disease is, the more important is this Rule Number 10. Just because your physician does not mention to you some new option you've heard about doesn't mean that new option does not have merit. Your doctor might not even know about it! Keep your eyes and ears open. Be aggressive in asking questions of your doctors, in presenting information to your doctors. After all, that's all part of your taking charge, taking ownership, in the management of your own chronic disease.

RULE NUMBER 11: Accept your chronic disease as a part of your life rather than focusing on it as a barrier to your getting the most out of your life. Acceptance of a chronic disease is a major factor in improving your health status. Day-to-day living has many facets. Only *one* of those is your disease. Your disease should not be your primary focus. Instead, your family, friends, and activities should reign paramount. Although your disease will dictate certain parameters of your activities, by focusing on your environment you can enhance the enjoyment of your day-to-day experience. If you refrain from obsessing about your physical condition, you will be less likely to limit yourself functionally and emotionally. By looking at the glass half-full rather than half-empty, you can avoid many of the pitfalls—such as depression and isolation—that tend to plague individuals suffering from chronic diseases. In the history of human thought and perspective, the effectiveness of mind over matter has been demonstrated time and again.

RULE NUMBER 12: Attempt to find mental, emotional, and spiritual comfort through prayer, meditation, reading, and discussing your needs openly with family, friends, and/or clergy. Based on your core values and your basic personality, you will find the combination of modalities that works best for you in meeting your own mental, emotional, and spiritual needs. These modalities understandably will vary from one person to another. As a guide for you to discover and make use of these modalities that can become such positive forces in your daily life, I have advice in both the intellectual and spiritual arenas. *In the intellectual arena, I recommend that every chronic disease patient reach out and make use of reading, meditating, and interacting with others.* By doing this, you will stay more in tune with yourself, you will become more in tune with others, and you will, as I have emphasized earlier, remain mentally active and socially involved. With reading, put some thought into seeking out meaningful reading materials of your choice. As part of that, read material you already know you like; and also absorb some new, mind-expanding reading materials. With meditation, make sure you allow time for periods of meditation in a suitable environment. It's not only important that you have time alone to reflect; it's also important that you do this in a setting that fits you. That might be in the den or on the porch of your home, it might be during a walk in your neighborhood or in the woods, or it could be in some other "special place." And, finally in the intellectual area, we come to the subject of interacting with others. I feel that interacting with others is so vital that I want to elaborate here on what I've already said about it in Rule Number 9, relative to avoiding isolation. As you structure your life to allow for interaction with others, it's important that you create opportunities to engage in stimulating discussions with as diverse a mixture of people as possible. This should include new people you bring into your life as well as longtime friends and family with whom you enjoy similar and often shared backgrounds.

When you're having discussions with others, explore the meaning of events that have occurred in your own life; but also make sure you take time to listen to others talk about their experiences, opinions, and advice. In thinking about those to involve in your discussions, consider including family, friends, new acquaintances, your physician, and members of the clergy. *In the spiritual arena, I would advise that you as a chronic disease patient make sure you do not focus so much on your disease that you neglect your spiritual needs.* For you to be the best you can be physically, it is extremely important that you are comfortable with and in tune with your spirituality. The spiritual path of choice will vary from one individual to another. For many, this path will include more prayer sessions. For some, the path will include an active searching, exploring, reaching out. For those who already have a strong faith and enjoy a personal relationship with God, the path often will involve increased consultations with a faith-based representative—a priest, rabbi, or minister; a lay church leader; or perhaps a faith-based physician or some other trusted spiritual counselor. As you follow your own spiritual path, it's important that you deal with a spiritual adviser who not only has your trust but also has the ability to advise you properly. Remember, now that you are waging a battle against chronic disease it becomes more important than ever that you reach outside yourself for spiritual comfort.

6

ATTENTION, PHYSICIANS: THERE ARE HOLES TO FILL!

Beginning back in my earlier days of practicing medicine, I began to be concerned about what I felt were some holes in our healthcare system in terms of how we address the ongoing care of patients suffering from chronic diseases.

Since I was diagnosed in 1995 with a chronic disease—myasthenia gravis—I've become even more convinced that these holes existed then and still exist today. I think we as a national medical community need to get busy filling some of these holes.

A Hole in Coordinating Care for the Chronic Disease Patient

A glaring hole that we have in our system—one prevalent with all chronic diseases—is that often there is no one in the healthcare field who's serving as the "medical quarterback" to manage the patient's chronic disease.

Often a chronic disease patient ends up with several physicians treating him or her, but with no one single physician who is in charge. A typical scenario is that the patient will be treated by one primary-care doctor and several specialists. Yet among all these physicians there's no one sitting at "central control." This means no one physician is functioning as medical traffic cop, keeping track of all the medical care the patient receives, and guiding the patient through the system. What happens unfortunately is that the primary-care physician who is supposed to be quarterbacking the patient's care often becomes just the one who is ping-ponging the patient from doctor to doctor. There is no consistent repository for data concerning an individual patient. This leads to duplication of testing and thus to increased cost. Also, there is no one physician who is fully informed about the patient.

This hole becomes a very relevant one because it's common for a chronic disease patient to suffer from multiple-system diseases that require multiple doctors. For the good of the patient and the management of his chronic disease, it's imperative that medical care rendered by various physicians be coordinated.

What problems have created this hole—this absence of the medical quarterback?

One of the problems is simply the super-specialized way our healthcare has come to be structured. We have become more focused on parts of the patient's body than on the patient as a whole. Beginning several decades ago, much of society's "doctoring" became more focused on systems than on the entire body; much of medical care became focused on the cardiovascular system, the gastrointestinal system, and other individual body systems. As the decades have gone by, we have become even more subspecialized. Now a patient's medical care often tends to be even more narrowly focused than it was 10 years ago. Today the focus often does not even extend to entire body systems, but instead is broken down into individual organs of the body. For example, often now the focus won't be on the gastrointestinal system as a whole; it's more like looking at the esophagus, or the stomach, or the gallbladder, or the intestines, all separately. On the one hand, there's a positive here in that this subspecialization has been fueled by the rapidly growing body of knowledge about each organ. Medical science just knows more today, and all that knowledge in one specialty category can't rest with one practitioner. On the other hand, it behooves physicians to take extra strides to work together more closely as a medical team, to make sure the patient's overall medical needs are being addressed. We also must make sure we are communicating with one another about a patient's care. If several doctors are treating the same patient, each of those doctors must be aware of what the other doctors are doing for this patient—including what medications each is prescribing. Too, the patient must be in this communication loop; physicians must make sure the patient understands what's going on in his care.

The reimbursement system represents another problem that has created this "hole." For years now the healthcare reimbursement system has not been structured to fairly compensate primary-care doctors for the often extensive amount of time required to serve as medical quarterback for a chronic disease patient. This picture is further complicated by the fact that we're talking about large numbers of patients; there are tremendous numbers of chronically ill patients who need a lot of physician time, attention, and coordination. The reimbursement system simply is not set up to give physicians such as family practitioners and internists the financial incentive to manage chronic illness as it should be managed. This unfair reimbursement system is widespread. It exists in federal healthcare payments to doctors via programs such as Medicare and Medicaid. It exists in health insurance programs such as the Blue Crosses and Blue Shields. And it exists in health maintenance organizations and preferred provider organizations, or PPOs. Throughout the 1980s, I felt the frustration of trying to address this inequity during my service in national organized medicine circles. I delved into this inequity in my roles as a member of the House of Delegates of the American Medical Association (AMA), vice chairman of AMA's Council on Medical Service, chairman of that council's Subcommittee on Financing Healthcare for the Elderly, and also chairman of the Task Force on Healthcare Financing and Reimbursement for the American College of Obstetricians and Gynecologists.

So what do we do in light of our tendency to have a super-specialized healthcare structure that often leaves the patient out in left field? And what do we do in light of the reality that the patient needs a medical quarterback but the reimbursement system isn't structured to fairly compensate a physician to do that job?

We do three things:

Number 1, we continue to refine our healthcare system so that the specialization becomes an enabler rather than an obstacle in addressing the needs of the typical chronic disease patient.

Number 2, we continue to peck away at reimbursement inequities by working through our medical organizations and in the political arena, making contacts with our congressmen and legislators and others who have the power to bring about change.

However, we don't wait until Number 1 and Number 2 are rectified before we join hands immediately in accomplishing *Number 3*—that is, putting together effective palliative-care programs in this nation to meet the needs of chronically ill patients.

Setting Up a Quality Program of Palliative Care

Before we even begin to address the goal of developing a quality palliative-care program, we need to think carefully about the very meaning of palliative care. The term "palliative" means "to ease without curing."

When we look at that meaning, we must realize that we're talking about bonding for the long haul with patients who have debilitating, often disabling, health problems. In rendering palliative care to a patient, the physician usually is dealing with a patient's health problem or problems for which there are only treatments and not cures. To effectively render this palliative care for the chronically ill requires knowledge on the part of the physician; it also calls for the physician to possess patience and caring. Quite frankly, I have seen some physicians become so frustrated with managing chronic disease that they would tend to withdraw and view the care as a burden rather than a privilege. It takes a special physician with a special attitude to take on any doctoring role for a patient in a palliative-care program. This holds true regardless of whether that physician is a primary-care doctor who treats the patient for decades or a specialist who is called in for short-term consultation.

I have four suggestions for the structure of a palliative-care program for chronic disease patients. And I have seven suggestions on how physicians should approach their roles in caring for chronic disease patients via a palliative-care program.

These are my four suggestions for the structure of a palliative-care program:
  • **The palliative-care program for the chronic disease patient should use a team approach.** It should usually be led by a primary-care

physician serving as medical quarterback, and should be supported by specialty physicians involved in the care of the patient. The medical quarterback physician usually would be an internist, a general practitioner, or a gerontologist. However, the medical quarterback might well be someone such as a rheumatologist or an endocrinologist or an obstetrician-gynecologist. A word of caution here: Never forget that the patient and the patient's primary caregiver are important members of this team.

- **Make sure all the needed physician resources have been called in to address this patient's multi-problems.** Typically, a chronic disease patient needs a wide range of medical support. For example, if a patient has diabetes and needs diabetic management, he might also have kidney problems and need a nephrologist, and could have heart problems and need a cardiologist, and could have eye problems and need an ophthalmologist. If a patient has rheumatoid arthritis, his primary doctor could be a rheumatologist. However the rheumatologist might need to call in an orthopedist, he might need to call in a cardiologist, and he might need to call in an endocrinologist. *But always, there must be a medical quarterback.*

- **Make sure that all the needed non-physician healthcare issues are addressed with the patient or caregiver—issues such as at-home care, support for the family, counseling services, etc.** Sometimes a primary-care doctor will want to raise these questions personally. Sometimes he assigns some of these tasks to an "extender" such as his nurse, a nurse practitioner, a physician's assistant, or a social worker. The important goal is that nothing should fall between the cracks. For the medical quarterback, this means not only serving as traffic cop among all the patient's doctors; it also means making sure the social issues and at-home care issues are addressed. Someone must ask the patient or his caregiver the right questions: "Do you have the community resources you need? Are you set up at home to give the care that's needed? Do you have access to all your medicines? In the event the caregiver can't support the patient, is there a family member or a friend on whom you can call?" And those are just samplings. In this book, I'm emphasizing that a patient or the patient's caregiver should assume ultimate responsibility for overall management of the patient's chronic disease. However, the reality of the situation is that the medical quarterback of a palliative-care team must be prepared to help the patient who can and does assume responsibility for his disease, as well as the patient who for some reason does not accept that responsibility.

• **Know about and work closely with resources in the community that can help the chronically ill patient.** The physician who serves as medical quarterback, or his extender, should be prepared to tell the patient or caregiver about community resources that can help with issues such as spiritual counseling, psychological counseling, home-healthcare, financial assistance, etc.

These are my seven suggestions for the approaches that all physicians in a palliative-care program should use in dealing with chronically ill patients. These suggestions are aimed not only at the physician who heads the palliative-care team as medical quarterback, but all other physicians who participate as well:

• **Look at the patient as your friend first and as your patient second.** Treat this patient as you would treat a member of your family—your wife or husband, your daughter or son. If you are considering recommending a surgical procedure or a new regimen of medicines for a patient, ask yourself, "Is this a treatment I would want used on my loved one under similar circumstances?" Also, through a caring manner and other means of communication—such as eye contact, a smile, and questions that show concern—show your patients the respect and love they deserve.

• **Listen to your patient.** I learned this in medical school from one of my professors, internationally acclaimed internist Dr. Tinsley Harrison, who authored a textbook on internal medicine that still is used in medical schools around the nation. Dr. Harrison always said that if you listen very closely to your patients, more often than not the patients will tell you what's wrong with them. I've seen this proven true so many times in dealing with patients. Yes indeed, a patient can help you with the diagnosis.

- **Let the patient know you're interested in him and his healthcare.** When I headed Henderson & Walton Women's Center in Birmingham, Alabama, the practice grew to 15 physicians; now that practice has 18 physicians. As my colleagues and I worked together in that large practice, we took special steps to ensure we were rendering patient care that was personalized, and care that was recognized by the patients as being personalized. Telephone calls to check on patients between office visits—phone calls placed by one of our nurses—let our patients know we were interested and also allowed us to stay current on what we needed to know to take care of the patient. Keeping in touch will improve your medical management of the patient. Keeping in touch also will let the patient know that you as his doctor still have him "on your radar screen."

- **Be honest with your chronic disease patients and with their caregivers by walking that fine-line balance of accuracy, reality, and hope.** Be realistic with the patient and the caregiver, while painting as positive a picture as you can. Trust in one's physician is essential in people who have chronic diseases and particularly in the case of uniformly fatal diseases. Most people can more easily accept devastating news if it is delivered in an honest, straightforward manner. Not destroying hope is the fine line that a physician must walk when communicating with the patient and caregiver. There is always something that can be offered, regardless of the severity of the patient's condition.

- **Fully and willingly accept your role of responsibility in caring for this chronically ill patient, without viewing it as a burden.** From time to time, stop and look at what's going on entirely from the patient's point of view. That view could be a real eye-opener. For example, let's consider here the medical care needs of a patient suffering from asthma. And for purposes of discussion, let's assume this patient is a young female—for there are indeed a lot of young females out there suffering from asthma. If you're the primary-care doctor for a young woman with asthma, what this young woman needs is palliative care to help her deal not only with the ravages of the asthma itself, but also the side effects of the treatments. She must deal with often devastating side effects of treatments such as steroids, plasmapheresis, and immunoglobulins. I've seen all too many young women suffering from asthma, and what I've seen them face is like a sort of unspoken devastating malignancy. While asthma is not a cancer per se, it can be compared with one in terms of the ruthlessness of the disease. Asthma is only one of many diseases that require a major commitment from the physician over a long period of time.

- **Individualize the treatment plan for every single chronic disease patient.** There's a great need for physicians to treat chronic disease patients as individuals, not with a cookie-cutter approach. Don't put every patient with the same diagnosis on a standard treatment regimen. Avoid going overboard in using standard templates. The approach of "one size fits all" is not a good one in managing healthcare for chronically ill patients. I know that since I have had myasthenia gravis, for example, I've become graphically aware that all autoimmune diseases are what I call "snowflake diseases." Just as no snowflakes are the same, just as no fingerprints are the same, just as no retinal images are the same, then no cases of myasthenia gravis or multiple sclerosis are the same. The same also extends to other chronic diseases.

- **Stay current with the scientific literature.** Needless to say, we are in an explosive age of knowledge. As a physician you owe it to your patients, and to yourself and other members of the palliative-care team, to stay abreast of the latest developments in your area of expertise.

A Hole in Diagnosing Chronic Disease

As a patient who has been diagnosed with myasthenia gravis, or MG, I would be remiss not to include a few words about the need for physicians to be alert and thorough in diagnosing chronic diseases.

While I am using MG as an example of how easy it is to miss a diagnosis, what I have to say here applies to many other chronic diseases as well.

My basic message: Be alert, listen to your patient, and don't be hesitant to think out of the box and to call in other specialists if you don't know what's wrong with a patient.

Myasthenia gravis is rare—only about 14 diagnosed patients per 100,000 population. It's a kind of "shadow disease"—unpredictable in the way it presents itself, causing one set of muscle-weakness and fatigue symptoms in one patient and quite a different set in another patient. Early on, prior to diagnosis, when MG victims have gone to doctors complaining of unusual feelings of fatigue and weakness, oftentimes their doctors have just dismissed the symptoms as being related to something going on in the patients' lives at the time. In some cases, the doctors have decided these patients were suffering from something vague such as chronic fatigue syndrome. And, sadly and unfortunately, some 60 percent of women who ultimately are diagnosed with MG are referred to psychiatrists before they get sent to neurologists.

Not only with MG, but with any set of patients' symptoms, physicians in general need to be aware of a wider range of potential diagnoses than can fit into what we call a "differential diagnosis" inventory. How do we accomplish that? I think it all comes down to opening our minds and broadening our horizons through increased awareness.

We who are taking the lead in spreading the word about MG need to make sure that practicing physicians, and also medical students and residents still in training, are made more aware of the symptoms of MG. And those who are taking the lead with other chronic diseases need to do the same—regardless of whether those diseases are rare or prevalent.

In the case of myasthenia gravis, it's such a rare disease that many primary-care physicians go their entire careers without ever seeing a case. Those who do see some cases are more likely to see the patients who have the eye-related MG—the ocular MG that causes symptoms such as double vision or drooping eyelids. A small percentage of primary-care doctors run across the more generalized form like I have, which causes muscular weakness in various parts of the body.

And, as for information about chronic diseases that is taught in medical school and residency, sometimes that information is very limited and
compressed. Since we are in an age where there is such a robust explo-
sion in knowledge, there is so little time to teach and so much to learn.
Myasthenia gravis is so rare that the amount of information included
about it in standard medical texts is very minimal. That's also true of
many other rare chronic diseases.

If I were going to give a piece of advice to doctors when it comes to
diagnosis in general, I would say don't fall into the trap of relying too
much on just what you've seen in your medical practice. If you're looking
across your desk at a patient in your office who has symptoms you don't
understand, the options of what's wrong with that patient do not neces-
sarily begin and end with the diagnoses you have seen over the years. I
think that's a big problem in the practice of medicine these days: That
problem is when making difficult diagnoses doctors often tend to rely
too much on their own experience, on their own databases, rather than
going back to the literature and/or calling in some help.

All in all, one thing is for sure: No matter how good a palliative-care
program you might set up, its outreach is limited if it's not serving the
patients who need it. The first step in helping a chronic disease patient
through a palliative-care program is to diagnose the patient properly
and make sure he's in the program that matches what's wrong with him.

Making the Most of Technology

In the age of modern-day technology, today's physicians have at their
disposal phenomenal technological tools to aid in the diagnosis and
treatment of patients suffering from chronic diseases.

By using the computer and the Internet, physicians can enhance
significantly the amount they can accomplish for patients and the ease
and speed with which they get it done.

Physicians can set up websites to which patients can go for information,
including results of laboratory and x-ray studies. They can use technology
to communicate rapidly with other physicians, to consult on numerous
patient-related issues. Physicians can use technology to connect them

with hospitals and clinics, pharmacists, medical equipment companies, and indeed with virtually all segments of the healthcare system.

Depending on how deeply involved a physician chooses to become with technology, other exciting options also are available. It's possible to have programs set up that allow for real-time video and audio conferencing with other physicians, related to consultation, training, continuing education, and other purposes. Too, some physicians have technological programs set up that enable them and/or members of their staffs to communicate directly with patients. This can be done in real time through options such as chat rooms and also in less time-sensitive forums such as message boards.

When physicians open the door to virtual communication, they unleash the power of a versatile tool that can extend their power to reach many audiences.

For the chronic disease patient who sits at his home computer and goes to a website set up by his doctor, the technology can become a vital bridge. Without making a special trip to the doctor's office, this patient can use his home computer to feel connected to his doctor. Seated in the comfort of his own home as he reads information on his doctor's website, the patient can learn more about his chronic disease, find out about new programs that might help him, and be alerted to other websites and articles that could inform him further. So long as a patient or his caregiver has access to a computer, I can envision very few circumstances in which this type of connector would not be both feasible and constructive. And, for chronically ill patients whose health problems often tend to isolate them and confine them to their homes much of the time, using the computer as a connector could become an especially valuable outlet.

For physicians who decide to use computerized technology to communicate with one another, this method of communication can enhance their ability in several areas. It can increase their ability to participate in doctor-to-doctor consults. It can aid doctors in their participation as members of multi-physician teams working together to diagnose and/or treat patients. By using e-mail to communicate with other doctors, a physician often can accomplish more in less time, and at more convenient times in the day, than with the use of phone calls, memos, letters, or in-person communication. And, via real-time video and audio conferencing, it can become possible for physicians who often are many miles apart to see and talk to one another without ever leaving their offices.

I challenge each and every physician in the United States to become computer literate to the extent of becoming as capable in using the computer and Internet as he or she is in diagnosing and treating patients.

7

A Caring, Competent Caregiver: A True Gift

I view good caregivers as being heroes. They indeed are the unsung, un-identified, and often, even in the view of the individual patients they're helping, unappreciated heroes in this society.

The primary caregiver for a patient holds tremendous powers in terms of how well the patient does emotionally and physically. As a physician I have seen many a case in which there was no doubt the primary caregiver made a difference in helping the patient to live a better quality of life and perhaps also a longer life.

The Importance of a Positive Attitude

The attitude of a patient's caregiver usually is directly transferable to the patient. If you find a primary caregiver who is negative and complain-ing, you tend to see that same attitude in the patient. On the flip side of that, if you have a positive, can-do person who is the primary caregiver and a major influence with that patient, this can lift the patient's spirits significantly.

I have seen positive primary caregivers do wonders in motivating even very sick chronically ill patients, even severely disabled patients with major challenges. I have seen positive caregivers actually empower patients with the ability to smile, the ability to embrace the good in life, the ability to climb over the next hill and not be totally demoralized and emotionally paralyzed.

This places a big responsibility on the shoulders of the primary care-giver to try to maintain a consistently positive attitude in the presence of the patient, even during times when the caregiver might not feel that positive attitude. If the caregiver does pass depressive feelings to the patient, those feelings can prove detrimental to the patient's health. The patient's maintaining of a positive attitude is relevant in terms of how well he does in coping with his disease. In short, the patient's attitude in turn often impacts how well he does mentally and physically. Negative breeds negative; and negative in a patient who has a chronic disease or disability, or both, can lead to further disability or even premature death.

Shouldering Heavy Loads

There are instances in which the responsibility placed on the shoulders of the caregiver is almost too huge and unrelenting to fathom.

Many heart-rending examples come to my mind. I particularly think of several women I've known who have given birth to babies with severe congenital problems. I have seen cases in which babies were born with problems so severe their mothers took care of the afflicted children for decades, sometimes for the rest of the mothers' lives. Among the more poignant of these situations involve mothers of severely mentally challenged Down syndrome children—children who can live into adulthood, to be 40 to 60 years of age, and never have the ability to take care of themselves. This is a tremendous load for the mothers who often are the primary and sometimes sole supporters for these individuals. For these mothers this represents a lifetime commitment. It requires a giving, a devotion, an unselfishness that is not recognized by the public in general.

Another example of a situation that requires extensive commitment on the part o the caregiver is support for the paralyzed patient—particularly the quadriplegic. It's not unusual for these patients to require minute-to-minute care. Unless there are resources available and unless there is a loving caregiver, these patients go unattended. The well-cared-for quadriplegic, for example, is going to live almost a normal lifespan. In fact, I have seen data indicating that the life span of a well-cared-for quadriplegic is only 10 years shorter than a normal lifespan. By contrast, the uncared-for quadriplegic is going to have a premature death because he's going to get skin ulcers or bed sores, he's going to get pneumonia, and he's going to get septicemia. The caregiver is all-important in making a difference.

Learning about the Patient's Health Problems

It's imperative that a primary caregiver learn as much as possible about the patient's particular health problem or problems.

If you as the caregiver do not understand the patient's health problem, or health problems, it's difficult to know how to interact with the patient and support him. If you don't understand, you will be more likely to view the situation as a burden. If you don't understand, you can't accept the situation and even embrace it as a challenge.

Too, if you don't understand the patient's health problems, you are limited in your ability to help care for the patient. You need insight into the patient's disease, illness, or injury to equip yourself to provide health maintenance support. For example, if the patient is a diabetic and tends to experience "lows" and "highs" with blood sugar, the caregiver must know how to intervene in those crises. If the patient takes various medications, the caregiver must be informed about these medications and their interactions.

Another reason the caregiver needs to understand the patient's health problems is to understand the emotional and lifestyle issues that are involved. In order to understand the patient's moods, concerns, and limitations, the caregiver must understand how the various health problems are impacting the patient. For example, my wife and children have become experts on my disease, myasthenia gravis, or MG. I know of many other myasthenics whose family members also have become very knowledgeable. They understand that MG is a cyclic disease, characterized by exacerbations and remissions. They understand that the myasthenic can feel great one morning but have difficulty getting out of bed the next. They know that some days are great, and that on other days it's like there is heavy weight attached to every part of the body. Myasthenia gravis is just an example. Each chronic disease has its own set of individual challenges. The caregiver must be tuned in to those challenges.

Communicating with the Patient's Physicians

If you are a caregiver who has major responsibilities in supporting a patient, it's crucial that you have a good line of communication with the patient's primary-care physician and with any other physicians involved in his care.

These physicians must understand the role you play in supporting the patient. You need to get to know these physicians and key contacts in their offices. You must receive ongoing information from the doctors regarding current issues in the patient's healthcare management. In addition, you must arrange in advance to have quick access to the doctors in times of emergency.

When you need additional resources from out in the community, you must speak up and ask the physicians and their staffs to assist you in locating these resources.

If you and the patient cannot communicate well with these physicians, you need to straighten out the communication problems or change physicians.

Researching and Accepting Help

A caregiver can greatly extend his or her ability to help the patient by taking inventory of help that's available and being willing to accept that help.

If you're shouldering the responsibility as the caregiver, it's important to both you and the patient that you not wear yourself out, that you not become physically and emotionally exhausted. You need rest periods yourself, away from the patient and the responsibilities.

Researching sources of help is one of the first things you should do after you find yourself in the role of a caregiver. If you don't feel comfortable conducting that research, you should assign the task to someone you trust to do a good job.

Even the most knowledgeable caregiver often is pleasantly surprised to identify the availability of helpful community resources about which he or she was unaware.

Make a list of the possible kinds of help you think you might need.

Then talk to a professional in the health field to expand that list of possibilities. Conduct research on who does the best job in various areas. And line up phone numbers and contacts even if you don't need these resources yet and might never need them. For example, as it relates to your situation, find out about home-healthcare, housekeeping assistance, health equipment rental, sitters, and therapy centers.

Include the spiritual and emotional side. Think out how you want to handle consulting with a minister, rabbi, priest, or any other representative of your faith. At least know where you can go for various types of counseling.

Don't put your family and friends at arm's length. Instead, talk candidly to them about your situation. Find out where they are willing and able to help, and avail yourself of that help. If you don't need the help currently, put your family members and friends on notice that you would like to call upon them when you do need help.

If you have a vacuum, a perceived need, that is not being filled, and if you don't know where to turn to meet that need, ask the patient's primary-care physician and his or her staff to advise and guide you.

Support Groups

Caregivers and patients have a wide range of views in how they feel about participating in support groups that relate to the patient's health problem, or health problems. For some patients and caregivers, it's a source of comfort and mutual support to interact with others who are in similar circumstances. To other patients and caregivers, it can be depressing.

Some of the more comprehensive support groups provide a wide range of services and interactions. I would advise any caregiver to at least look at relevant support groups and take stock of what they have to offer. You might or might not want to sit around in support group meetings and exchange stories about healthcare issues. However, you might find that you learn valuable information from speakers at a group's meetings. You might find that members of the support group can help you with problems and that you in turn can help them. Also, you might find it uplifting to join with members of a group in programs aimed at helping other patients and their families.

Support groups are worthy of your investigation.

A Tribute to a Special Caregiver

I know I am greatly blessed in that my primary caregiver during two health-related crises in my life has been one of the most unselfish people on the face of the earth—my wife, Beth.

Beth always has been my chief supporter, ever since our marriage 44 years ago when I was weeks away from 21 and she was still 19. She has done a tremendous job in supporting me professionally, in maintaining our household, and in nurturing our three children, Rhonda, Ellen, and Bill.

However, since I was blessed with excellent health and incredible stamina, Beth was never placed in a major care-giving role with me until December 1974. That was when I was involved in a car accident and sustained severe injuries. I was hospitalized for weeks, and then I was involved in rehabilitation before and after I returned to work much earlier than my doctors had hoped for or predicted. During this period in 1974 and 1975, I was afforded a memorable firsthand glimpse into what a life-changing event a health crisis can be for a family—particularly for the primary caregiver, in this case my beautiful Beth. After I had my accident, Beth was always there for me. Friends reached out to help us with the children. Beth was there at my side at the hospital from sunrise until sundown daily. She was at my side supporting me and taking care of me after she brought me home from the hospital. Then she was there driving me to my rehabilitation sessions and also to my office to return to work. Beth was incredible. As bad as that accident was in many ways, it turned out to be a positive event for my life. I learned a lot, and it was unifying for Beth and me in our marriage. While I'm sorry that it happened, there's no doubt the event proved to be a positive in leading me toward a more in-depth insight into the meaning of my life and my missions in life. Because of that accident, I feel that I became a better physician, a better husband and father, and a better human being.

Then, in 1994, after I began showing mysterious symptoms ultimately diagnosed in November 1995 as being caused by myasthenia gravis,

Beth and I were introduced to what it was like to live with a chronic, incurable disease. We knew that what we faced together now was not an acute event such as my 1974 wreck, but instead a chronic situation. My wreck involved several consecutive months of life disruption, if you add up the weeks of my hospital stay plus the period of rehabilitation that followed. However, after I was diagnosed with myasthenia gravis, we had an ongoing battle on our hands. We were facing the prospect of living a lifetime managing a chronic disease that at least for now is not curable. Today I am of course continuing to deal with this disease, and will continue to deal with it until if and when a cure is found. I'm on top of managing my disease and feeling well enough to be active and to reach out to help others. However, on my darkest days during my early MG period, I was combating not only myasthenia gravis but also periodic bouts with asthma and bronchitis. During those times, I was spending most of my time in bed, and taking my meals in bed. Over a period of months, there was a lot of time when I didn't want to have to get up or even get on the phone. Oftentimes when I wasn't taking my meals in the bed, I was taing them in my recliner; and Beth would bring the meals to me. Beth also did all the extender work to keep the household going, and she was doing all the driving. I never got to the point where I had to be fed. However, I was so weak Beth had to help me with tasks such as buttoning my shirts and removing tops from bottles. (She *still* helps me at times with those kinds of tasks!)

Through it all, Beth has never complained. And our three children and son-in-law and daughter-in-law also have reflected that positive attitude. All the family has been absolutely wonderful. And Beth has been the leader, the core of support.

As I watched Beth support me through very difficult times, it seemed to me that she never viewed what she was doing as a burden. I think she looked upon it as her duty and her responsibility. Also, I think she viewed being a support to me as almost a challenge, which she met in spades. She did it lovingly, and I think she received satisfaction out of doing it well.

There is no doubt in my mind that I would never have come this far without Beth's support, without her awesome strength, and without her positive spirit.

To me, Beth Summerville Henderson possesses all the qualities of a competent, caring caregiver. She continues to demonstrate those qualities every single day.

8

Communities, Rise to the Challenge!

Never before in the history of our society has there been a more pressing need for community programs to help chronically ill patients and their caregivers.

At the same time, it is my opinion that the majority of communities in this nation are falling far short in establishing and operating such programs.

I think the basic reason for this is that there is a trend in the United States toward the disappearance of community cohesiveness—the type of cohesiveness that decades ago led citizens within a given community to come together to do good. Oh, there are shining lights of exceptionality. But in general we are tending to lose what I call the "matrix" of our communities, the core of our community spirit.

Gradually over the past several decades, America on the whole has evolved into an increasingly individualistic society marked by community residents living lives that are fast-paced, self-absorbed, and detached. Add to that the transient nature of our communities—so many people coming and going without making meaningful connections, without putting down roots. Add further the trend for millions of Americans to work in one city or town and live in another, spending a significant portion of their days commuting back and forth between the two locations and never really connecting to either.

When it comes to communities stepping forward to meet the needs of the chronically ill and their caregivers, it's ironic that some of the very factors that create a bigger need for services also can create barriers to setting up those services. For example, look at the transient nature of our society. There are many chronically ill patients who have moved into communities from distant locations and have fallen victim not only to chronic health problems but also to isolation. Many have no relatives living nearby to aid with caregiving for their chronic health problems, and many have become so preoccupied with their health problems that they have not made friends in the community. The irony of this situation is that the transient makeup of many communities also often forms a barrier that prevents community residents from getting to know one another and coming together to set up and operate programs to aid the chronically ill.

I do think there are solutions. But in order for any of these solutions to take root and bear fruit, at least one "doer" in the community has to take an interest. That person needs to be caring, aggressive, productive, and creative. It helps if that individual has a few other interested helpmates who have the same traits.

The First Step: Taking Inventory

Communities differ greatly in structure and focus. However, I dare say there is not a single community in America that cannot greatly improve upon its community support services to aid chronically ill patients and their caregivers.

The first step in making these improvements is to take inventory of the programs that exist and to take inventory of the people who need help.

As those inventories emerge, it will become clear where gaps exist in programs, and where gaps exist in making sure that programs reach the people who need them.

A word of caution here: Funds to support these types of programs are too scarce and precious to duplicate programs unnecessarily. Dating back to the days in the 1970s when I was involved in health planning, I have been an advocate of sharing community social service and health programs. Your community might want to join with several other surrounding communities to create a much-needed program to serve the chronically ill. Or if your community is located near a city that already has a relevant program, you might want to focus your attention on creating a transportation service to transport your citizens to and from that neighboring program.

What Kinds of Programs Are Needed?

Patients who are chronically ill need a variety of services. What one patient needs another might not need.

If you were to study the needs of 100 chronically ill patients and their caregivers, I would venture to say that most all would need medical care and transportation to and from doctors' offices, clinics, and hospitals. Some will have those needs covered, but many will not.

Some percentage of those 100 chronically ill patients and their caregivers would have unmet needs in the following additional areas plus many more:

- Spiritual counseling
- Psychological counseling
- Financial assistance
- Housing assistance
- Medical equipment rental or purchase
- Home health services
- Housekeeping services
- Sitter services and respite care to relieve the caregivers
- Assistance with errands such as grocery shopping and going to the drugstore
- Information and understanding will be a gap in the homes of many chronically ill patients. Many patients and caregivers simply need someone who is knowledgeable and patient enough to sit down and teach them about the disease or diseases with which they are dealing.
- There will be a small percentage that will need the services of nursing homes for chronically ill patients who cannot be managed at home.
- There will be some who will need hospice services for chronically ill patients in the terminal stages of illness and thus in the latter months and weeks of life.

• And, for many a patient and caregiver, there's a pressing need just for some caring people in the community to take a sincere interest and come by to visit—to show concern, bring a positive attitude, and ease the isolation.

Who Can Take the Lead in Running Community Programs?

As communities have become more fast-paced and detached, some of the agencies and civic organizations that once took a lead have disappeared.

However, some strongholds remain. I think as a general rule some of the biggest nominees to take a leadership role in community outreach are local churches and the YMCAs and YWCAs—the Young Men's Christian Associations and the Young Women's Christian Associations. I know the churches and the YMCA in particular still are extremely active in the community of Prattville, Alabama, where my wife, Beth, and I grew up and where we still maintain a second home. I see the good these organizations can do, and I believe they have "sister and brother" organizations across America that also can function as facilitators to do good.

In addition, there are foundations, associations, and support groups—each representing a health problem or group of health problems—that can play constructive roles. Some of these organizations have strong structures, far-reaching databases, and in some cases programs that already exist which could help many more people. I'm speaking of groups such as the Heart Association, Cancer Society, Myasthenia Gravis Foundation, Multiple Sclerosis Society, and Arthritis Foundation. There also are numerous support groups, representing a host of chronic health problems, which might not be affiliated with a health-related foundation or association. As a physician, I've seen many chronically ill people who could use the help of a support group but who don't participate because they are shy, modest, or reticent. Often some of these people just need an encouraging word from a member of one of these groups—to know the welcome mat is out and that help and support are available.

My Challenge to Individual Community Citizens

No matter how much our communities have changed, there still are individuals who live in those communities who want to reach out to touch and help others. The big difference in yesterday and today is that today it sometimes takes more effort to carve out the time to convert good intentions into good deeds.

In advocating that Americans carve out that time, President George W. Bush is telling all of us that through volunteerism we can make a tremendous impact.

I challenge you to remember that one person can make a difference. You could start by offering additional support to your friends and acquaintances who are dealing with chronic health problems—patients and their caregivers with whom you already feel comfortable and whom you feel could benefit from your love and support. If you know someone who is chronically ill, check on the needs of that person and the caregiver. Visit when you think it's appropriate. And offer to relieve the caregiver with assistance such as running an errand or sitting with the patient while the caregiver takes the afternoon off.

You have the power to lift up others, to relieve some stress, and to put some smiles on some faces. It truly is more blessed to give than to receive.

The Power of a Seed

I challenge communities across this nation to step forward to set up new programs to aid the chronically ill, to expand and/or revitalize old programs, and to take steps to see that these programs reach the patients and caregivers who need them.

The seed that is needed to do this will vary from community to community. In one community, it could be a wealthy individual who has money to invest in such a program but who needs help from community leaders who have talents in organization. In another community, it could be an organizer or organizers whose first step needs to be raising funds to do the job. And in still another community, the seed could be a local club or agency that is looking for a worthy project to help people and at the same time to unite the community.

In all cases, there must be a catalyst for change. That catalyst must be accompanied by a workable plan, follow-through, deadlines, and a contagious can-do spirit that spreads motivation and enthusiasm among all those who participate.

I want you to remember what a tremendous difference one person can make.

PART THREE

TREATING AND RESEARCHING
MYASTHENIA GRAVIS

Opening Doors to Treatment and Research of Myasthenia Gravis

This book focuses on myasthenia gravis from the viewpoint of individuals such as I, who actually are experiencing the disease. Also, this book looks at MG from the viewpoint of the physician who treats the disease and the researcher who is attempting to find new MG treatments and perhaps even a cure.

The following three chapters delve into some of the elements related to treatment and research.

To gain insight into the view of a physician who treats the disease, I spoke with neurologist Dr. Shin J. Oh. I consulted with Dr. Oh partly because I have personal reason to appreciate Dr. Oh's understanding of myasthenia gravis—for he has been involved in my own MG management the past several years. I also turned to Dr. Oh because he has decades of experience in treating MG patients and is internationally known for his work in the MG field.

To explore a promising project of MG research, I interviewed Dr. J. Edwin Blalock. At the present time, Dr. Blalock is involved deeply in research aimed at finding a vaccine that hopefully could cure MG—a vaccine that, if it proves effective, will be targeted for use in patients who already have the disease. A basic researcher, or bench scientist, with a Ph.D. in medical microbiology/immunology, Dr. Blalock has a sterling scientific record which for years has included research on problems related to the immune system, including MG.

Dr. Blalock is based in the Department of Physiology and Biophysics at the University of Alabama at Birmingham (UAB). Dr. Oh also is based at UAB, in the Departments of Pathology and Neurology at the University of Alabama School of Medicine. This is a medical school which enjoys an outstanding reputation and one in which I take particular pride, since it is my alma mater.

For an overview of other research projects in the MG area and related fields, I consulted the current literature and several scientists on the front lines.

I feel it appropriate to express gratitude to the dedicated clinicians such as Dr. Oh to whom MG patients turn for treatments to keep them healthy enough to enjoy today, and the brilliant researchers such as Dr. Blalock who in their hands hold the promise of tomorrow.

RONALD E. HENDERSON, M.D.

9

A Journey in the Treatment
of Myasthenia Gravis

As I sat and talked with Dr. Shin Oh about treatment options for patients with myasthenia gravis, Dr. Oh was like a fountain of information who could describe present-day treatments and also trace treatments of the past.

A full professor of both neurology and pathology, Dr. Oh today holds a string of appointments that speak to his internationally recognized expertise in areas such as myasthenia gravis and various neuropathies. It was in 1970 when Dr. Oh joined the medical school faculty at the rapidly growing and now renowned medical center based at the University of Alabama at Birmingham (UAB). He came there a decade after receiving his medical degree in his native Korea, a few years after finishing his residency at Georgetown University Hospital in Washington, D.C., and a couple of years after completing his research fellowship at the University of Minnesota Medical Center in Minneapolis. He was fresh off a faculty appointment at Meharry Medical College in Nashville, Tennessee.

As a young neurologist who quickly moved up the ladder of medical academia from assistant professor to associate professor, Dr. Oh found himself deeply involved in teaching and supervising neurology residents as they took care of patients suffering from a range of neurological problems. This included patients suffering from myasthenia gravis, or MG. He remembers well the difficulty in providing medical management for a seriously ill MG patient back in the 1970s.

It was such a different world then from what it is today in managing MG, explained Dr. Oh.

He said if a patient is diagnosed accurately with MG in the present-day era, and if that patient has access to quality treatment, the patient is in a much better position to be managed well than were MG patients of decades gone by.

Using Prednisone To Treat MG

Dr. Oh believes the biggest single factor accounting for improved management of the MG patient is expanded knowledge on how to safely and effectively use steroid medication—namely, prednisone—as a part of the MG treatment regimen.

"When I think back to the 1970s, I remember that in treating the MG patient we often had a fear that we would lose the patient, that the patient would die," said Dr. Oh. "I recall so many situations with hospitalized MG patients in which the patient was in crisis. And we would have to monitor the patients constantly day and night. Today we don't have much of the kind of grim or pessimistic situation that we had in the past with MG. Now if the MG patient has access to good care, the disease usually can be managed quite well. The biggest single difference between now and back then is that now we know how to treat the MG patients with the help of steroids. And we also know how to manage the patients so that we don't have to keep them on high dosages of steroids for so long. Back then we didn't have much experience in using high dosages of steroids."

As both a physician and a patient, I know it's so important that MG patients have a thorough understanding of the steroid medication known as prednisone, which virtually always is used to treat MG.

In treating severe cases of myasthenia gravis, it is essential that immunosuppressive drugs, including prednisone, be used to "put out the fire." By that I refer to the fact that in severe MG cases the body is producing large quantities of destructive antibodies that must be neutralized.

Just as I realize how important it is to use prednisone to treat the MG patient, I also feel it's imperative to discuss prednisone in detail—for two reasons. One reason relates to the power of prednisone to help the MG patient. Another reason concerns the power of prednisone to produce serious side effects and to place the patient at risk for developing other health problems.

On the one hand, prednisone can be very effective in helping the MG patient. Prednisone helps by suppressing the ability of the MG patient's immune system to produce damaging antibodies that cause the muscle weakness and fatigue associated with MG.

On the other hand, the side effects and risks associated with extensive use of prednisone are multiple in number and several of them serious in nature. The side effects can include mood swings (from depression to euphoria and back again), difficulty sleeping, hyperactivity, increased appetite, fluid retention, weight gain, thinning and bruising of the skin, and excessive hair growth. One ongoing risk in taking prednisone is that this medication can cause the patient to be more susceptible to infections, because the patient's immune system becomes suppressed to the degree it is less able to fight off outside invaders such as infections. Also, extensive use of prednisone can place the patient at risk for developing health problems such as high blood pressure, osteoporosis, cataracts, glaucoma, and steroid-induced diabetes.

When prescribing steroids, the physician must always weigh the benefit to the patient versus the adverse side effects caused by the drug.

The patient taking prednisone must be fully informed of the side effects and risks. Also, the patient who is taking prednisone must be monitored carefully by a knowledgeable, attentive physician. For example, the patient should be under the care of a physician who understands fully the necessity to refrain from ever taking the patient off prednisone suddenly. If a patient is coming off prednisone, he must taper off gradually. Otherwise, the patient can suffer serious withdrawal symptoms such as nausea, vomiting, and fever. Also, if a patient stops taking prednisone without tapering off properly, the patient can experience a sudden flare-up of the symptoms of whatever health problem led to his taking the prednisone in the first place. In the case of the MG patient, this would mean a flare-up of symptoms related to muscle weakness and fatigue.

Taking Aim at MG with a Range of Medications

While prednisone has played, and continues to play, a vital role in helping so many patients suffering from MG, it definitely is not the only medication being used to take aim at MG.

Dr. Oh and I discussed the various medications used to combat MG. We discussed how one type of medication attacks MG by one means, while another type of medication takes a totally different approach.

We also talked about MG itself and the reasons certain medications work as they do to combat it.

The way MG works actually is quite clearly understood—better understood than some other autoimmune diseases such as multiple sclerosis and Guillain-Barré syndrome. In fact, there are some in the immunology field who view MG as the best understood of all autoimmune diseases.

When a patient has MG, various muscles in his body become weak and fatigued because the patient's muscles cannot contract as they should. The muscles can't contract because there's an abnormal process going on in the MG patient's body—involving an abnormal antibody—that is preventing nerve impulses from being transmitted to muscles. The muscles must be able to receive these nerve impulses in order to contract.

In an individual who does not have MG, the nerve endings normally release a neurotransmitter substance called acetylcholine, and the muscle contracts after the acetylcholine activates some receptor sites. However, in the MG patient, the patient's overactive immune system is producing damaging antibodies that are destroying or blocking these acetylcholine receptor sites.

Many MG patients get help in combating this abnormal antibody activity by taking one or more medications in a category referred to as "immunosuppressants." These are medications that are used to treat a wide range of health problems by suppressing the immune system. In the case of the MG patient, the immunosuppressants are used to limit the body's ability to produce the damaging abnormal antibodies that block or destroy the acetylcholine receptor sites.

Then there's another type of medication available to the MG patient that does not interfere with production of abnormal antibodies. Instead, this type of medication is designed to increase muscle strength by maximizing the patient's access to this vital neurotransmitter substance called acetylcholine.

Dr. Oh outlined some of his own criteria in using these various medications to treat MG patients.

In using immunosuppressant medications to treat MG patients, Dr. Oh said there is no question that his first choice in this group is the steroid medication prednisone. However, he hastened to add that prednisone alone won't work for some MG patients. Dr. Oh said some patients need additional treatment that is selected from another choice of immunosuppressant medications. The immunosuppressant medications in this group include Imuran®, cyclosporine, CellCept®, and Cytoxan®. The first three on this list—Imuran®, cyclosporine, and CellCept®—are among immunosuppressants that have been used to treat organ transplant patients; these medications have been used to reduce the chances the patients' bodies will reject the transplanted organs. The other drug, Cytoxan®, has been used quite a bit as a chemotherapy agent to treat cancer patients.

As for the category of medication that works to increase the muscle strength of the MG patient without suppressing the immune system, this category often is called "anticholinesterase therapy." This type of medication is designed to increase muscle strength by improving neuromuscular transmission. The way this type of medication improves neuromuscular transmission is to prevent the breakdown of the vital neurotransmitter substance known as acetylcholine. The objective is for more of the acetylcholine to accumulate at the neuromuscular junction. This junction is where the nerve impulses interact with the muscles to bring about muscle contraction. A widely used medication that falls in this category is Mestinon®.

Dr. Oh said it is not uncommon for the main MG treatment regimen for a patient to consist of Mestinon® and also some type of immunosuppressant regimen, most often prednisone.

"When patients have generalized myasthenia gravis (MG affecting various parts of the body), my criteria is that if Mestinon® alone doesn't work, then these patients also are given immunosuppressive medication," said Dr. Oh.

Using Blood-Related Treatments for MG

When medications alone won't do the job in controlling the symptoms of a MG patient, Dr. Oh said he turns to one of two other treatments—both blood-related treatments. With some patients, he uses both of these treatments.

One of these treatments is IVIg. The other is plasmapheresis.

"If we have a myasthenia gravis patient who is facing a crisis situation, or even a patient who is not in a real crisis but is getting very weak, we tend to use the IVIg or the plasmapheresis," said Dr. Oh. "And if one does not work, we can turn to the other. For example, if the IVIg treatment is not effective, we would go ahead and use the plasmapheresis."

IVIg officially is intravenous immune globulin. Other terms by which it is known include "gamma globulin" or "pooled human gamma globulin." The IVIg is a product of human blood that has been donated by multiple donors—a blood product that is rich in antibodies. Over the years, IVIg has been used as a treatment to replace antibodies in patients fighting various infectious or inflammatory diseases. In the case of the MG patient, whose own body is producing some abnormal antibodies, the IVIg treatment temporarily provides the patient with normal antibodies. The IVIg treatment is administered to the patient intravenously. It is given slowly, sometimes over a period of hours and sometimes broken into a series of infusions.

As for the plasmapheresis, this is a procedure in which the plasma is removed from a MG patient's own blood, and then is replaced. It's replaced with fresh frozen plasma, a blood product called albumin, and/or a plasma substitute. In treating the MG patient with plasmapheresis, the goal is to remove abnormal antibodies from the patient's bloodstream.

Treating the MG Patient with Surgery

Quite a number of patients who are diagnosed with myasthenia gravis undergo a surgical procedure called "thymectomy."

A thymectomy is the surgical removal of the thymus gland. Located in the upper chest area beneath the sternum, or breastbone, the thymus gland plays a role in the immune system.

Somewhere around 10 percent of all MG patients are found to have a tumor of the thymus gland, called a thymoma. When a patient is diagnosed with a thymoma, unless there are extremely extenuating circumstances, a thymectomy generally is always recommended. This is done not only with the goal of reducing MG symptoms, but also as a precaution due to the risk of malignancy associated with the tumor.

In addition to a thymectomy being recommended for MG patients diagnosed with a thymoma, many MG patients who don't have a thymoma also undergo a thymectomy. They have the thymectomy as part of the treatment regimen designed to reduce MG symptoms. Dr. Oh believes a patient definitely does not have to be diagnosed with a thymoma in order to be considered a viable candidate for a thymectomy.

The thymectomy is major surgery. A patient needs to be fully informed and fully prepared prior to surgery, and the surgeon performing the thymectomy should be one who is knowledgeable and experienced in this particular surgery.

Dr. Oh said there are two groups of MG patients he generally excludes when it comes to recommending a thymectomy, unless there is a thymoma present. He excludes one group because of an age issue, and he excludes another group based on the type of MG that's involved. On the age factor, Dr. Oh said he does not recommend a thymectomy for MG patients who are older. Specifically, he said generally he does not recommend a thymectomy for anyone who is over age 65. The second group for whom he does not recommend a thymectomy is that group of patients who suffer from the form of MG that is limited to the eye area. This is "ocular MG"—a form of MG that affects only the eyes and/or eyelids and does not include muscle weakness in other parts of the body.

On a broad scale there's a wide range of experience among individual patients as to how much MG relief they get after undergoing thymectomy. This ranges from reports from patients who enjoy major remissions of MG symptoms to reports from patients who feel they get little symptom-relief benefit. However, Dr. Oh reported a high degree of symptom relief among his own MG patients who have undergone this surgery to remove the thymus gland.

Dr. Oh said in many situations he has seen thymectomy bring about significant relief for MG patients: "Generally I think the patients I've treated who have undergone the thymectomy procedure tend to do much better than those who do not. They tend to need a smaller number of drugs and less dosage of the drugs, and I've known of many who don't have to be managed on any medicine."

As for the timetable when patients can expect to start feeling MG symptom relief following thymectomy, this, too can vary quite a bit from patient to patient. For those patients who experience reduction in MG symptoms following a thymectomy, it is not uncommon for a good deal of time to pass before they start feeling the benefits. That could be months after surgery, a year after surgery, even longer.

Cost Issues

For many MG patients, the issues of treatment extend far beyond whether a particular treatment works or does not work for them. For many, there's a major issue also in how to pay for the treatments.

While some medications used to treat MG are relatively inexpensive, that's not the case for certain other medications.

Dr. Oh told me there are situations in which pharmaceutical company assistance has made it possible to get medications into the hands of medically needy MG patients who otherwise would not have had access. However, Dr. Oh said that all the needs in that area are far from being covered.

Also, Dr. Oh noted that one blood-related treatment used to treat myasthenia gravis—the IVIg, or intravenous immune globulin—runs into thousands of dollars per treatment and thus is out of reach for a large percentage of patients. "I know there aren't too many people in our state who could afford this treatment on an ongoing basis," said Dr. Oh.

All in all, said Dr. Oh, broadening patients' access to more of the MG treatments is definitely a need that should be addressed. "I think through opening up access to these medications for patients who are having difficulty obtaining them, this becomes an area of assistance which can be so directly helpful to specific MG patients," he said.

Diagnosing a Patient with MG

If a physician suspects that a patient could have myasthenia gravis, there are several diagnostic tools to help confirm or rule out this diagnosis.

The physician can inject into a patient's vein the chemical known as Tensilon®, also known as edrophonium chloride. If a patient is having MG symptoms, the Tensilon® can cause these symptoms to get much better quickly. Tensilon® is not used as an ongoing treatment for MG once it is diagnosed, because the improvement in MG symptoms using this chemical is really very temporary. However, Tensilon® can be an effective tool for diagnosis.

Also, as a part of his own diagnostic workup, Dr. Oh sometimes includes the medication Mestinon® that's used to treat MG. Again, just as with the Tensilon®, if the patient's muscle-weakness symptoms become conclusively better after taking Mestinon®, that can be an indication the patient has MG.

There also are blood studies that can be done—to look for the presence of immune molecules or abnormal antibodies associated with MG.

Some physicians also use electromyography as a part of a diagnostic workup related to MG. With electromyography, the physician uses equipment to stimulate muscle fibers with electrical impulses. By measuring how muscle cells react to the electrical impulses, a diagnostician can gain valuable information. If a patient has myasthenia gravis, his muscle fibers do not tend to respond to the electrical stimulation as well as the muscle fibers of an individual who does not have myasthenia gravis.

As Dr. Oh and I discussed issues related to diagnosing MG, our conversation turned to issues related to two groups of patients in particular.

With the first group, we were discussing those patients who have MG but who tend to go undiagnosed because doctors don't suspect this diagnosis and thus don't take steps to get the patients tested.

In the second group, we were discussing situations relevant to patients who report symptoms that sound like MG but who in reality do not have MG.

With the first group—the MG sufferers who often go so long without being diagnosed—vague symptoms often are a problem with diagnosis.

In the case of a patient who ultimately is diagnosed with MG, it's not unusual for that individual's first symptom to be simply one of fatigue, just feeling very tired. If this problem of fatigue is the only symptom the patient is feeling, and thus the only symptom the patient initially reports to his doctor, it then falls to the doctor to consider the various things that could be causing the tired feeling. And there are many possibilities. A symptom of chronic fatigue can relate to many different health conditions, and certainly not just to myasthenia gravis. That can be a tough diagnosis to make at that point. A patient could actually have myasthenia gravis but be at a point where the only real symptom he is noticing is chronic fatigue. He might not yet have reached the point where he's experiencing other symptoms that would more specifically point to myasthenia gravis—symptoms that include double vision, the difficulties chewing or swallowing, those kinds of things.

It's important that physicians be informed about the various symptoms associated with myasthenia gravis. If a physician is familiar with symptoms of MG, he can utilize this information as part of the knowledge base he employs when diagnosing certain patients. For example, when a patient comes in complaining of unexplained fatigue and/or various muscle-weakness symptoms, the physician can at least consider MG as an option to investigate. In fact, Dr. Oh feels that it's particularly important to provide ongoing MG information updates to primary-care physicians: "In targeting information about myasthenia gravis to physicians, it's important to alert particularly those physicians who tend to see the patient initially after the patient starts having symptoms. This includes the family physicians and the physicians in internal medicine."

Just as physicians need to be made aware of how not to miss a MG diagnosis, they must be made aware of how to avoid making an incorrect MG diagnosis, said Dr. Oh.

Dr. Oh said while he is aware there's a problem with under-diagnosis of MG, he's also aware that it's possible for a patient to be told he has MG when he doesn't have it. One way that can happen, he explained, is for a patient to read up on the symptoms of MG and be convinced he has the disease and report these symptoms to the doctor. Dr. Oh said if the diagnostician does not take precautions, he could think a diagnostic test is positive for MG when it is not. For that reason, Dr. Oh said he is careful to build into his own diagnostic workup some controlled studies that check and double-check. That way, Dr. Oh said there is a system of checks and balances in place to prevent a false MG diagnosis in a patient who incorrectly perceives he's getting muscle-weakness relief from agents such as Tensilon® or Mestinon®.

Advice to Myasthenia Gravis Patients

In the material that follows you will find four suggestions for patients who suspect they have myasthenia gravis or who have been diagnosed with myasthenia gravis. These suggestions include valuable input from Dr. Oh. They also include my observations as a MG patient—observations based on my own experiences with MG and on my interfacing with many other MG patients.

NUMBER 1. Involve a physician in your diagnosis and treatment who has specialized knowledge about myasthenia gravis. I believe a patient should involve a neurologist in investigating a possible diagnosis of MG and also in ongoing treatment of MG. Dr. Oh agreed, adding this explanation: "A neurologist is the physician who is trained in the medical specialty that includes the diagnosis and treatment of myasthenia gravis."

NUMBER 2. Educate yourself about myasthenia gravis. Again, as I have emphasized previously in this book, I believe it's important for a patient to take ownership of his or her chronic disease. And I feel this is particularly true of myasthenia gravis. Dr. Oh had this perspective: "I think educating yourself about your disease is such a very important thing to do. You really have to be inquisitive. Today patients are so much more self-educated about health problems than they were in decades past. However, I would add one word of caution. If you are the type of person who tends to imagine you have various types of health ailments, beware of going to the Internet and learning about MG and then going to the neurologist and reporting that you are feeling all those symptoms."

NUMBER 3. Be open in asking your physicians any questions that you have. Remember, as I already have emphasized, be assertive and even aggressive in communicating with your physician about your disease. Dr. Oh added: "Do not shy away from asking questions of your physician. You must be active for yourself in seeking information and answers."

NUMBER 4. Change physicians if you are not satisfied. I can see any number of reasons why a patient might feel a given physician is not the right one for him or her. The patient might have trouble establishing open communication with the physician. Or the patient might feel the care he or she is receiving is inadequate or not up to date. Dr. Oh had this advice: "There is no reason why you have to stick with one physician if you are not satisfied. If you feel the need, you have the right to disassociate yourself from a particular physician and to seek medical help elsewhere."

A Medical Expert's View of the MG Future

When Dr. Shin Oh began making his decision in the 1960s about which specialty to enter, he was headed toward a choice that was far from being mainstream. He selected neurology, which was not among the more commonly selected specialties. Then he went a step further and in a sense selected a subspecialty—neuromuscular diseases. These are diseases that have a relationship to the function of, and health problems related to, the muscles and nerves.

"At the time I went into this field, we didn't have too many neurologists who were interested in neuromuscular diseases," said Dr. Oh.

As he pursued his chosen field, Dr. Oh had access to excellent postgraduate education. He took extensive training in electromyography, the use of electrical activity for tasks that include diagnosis of various neuromuscular disorders. Too, Dr. Oh was among those to take training at the National Institutes of Health, under the direction of the noted neuromuscular disease expert Dr. King Engel.

As Dr. Oh developed his own international reputation over the years, he became known as an expert especially on two neurological disorders. One disorder about which he is considered highly knowledgeable is

CIDP; this is chronic inflammatory demyelinating polyneuropathy, a progressive weakness and sensory dysfunction of the arms and legs. Also, Dr. Shin Oh is considered an expert on myasthenia gravis.

Dr. Oh is the widely published author of numerous scientific articles, including articles on myasthenia gravis and myasthenic syndrome. He has been selected to serve on review boards for scientific publications such as the *American Journal of Medicine, Annals of Neurology, Muscle & Nerve,* and *Neurology.* He's the author of several books; among them is *Electromyography: Neuromuscular Transmission Studies.*

As for the academic and clinical appointments Dr. Oh holds today at UAB, they are multiple. In the medical school, he's a full professor of neurology and pathology. In the medical school's Department of Neurology, he's director of the Muscle and Nerve Histopathology Laboratory. At UAB's University Hospital, he's medical director of the Department of Clinical Neurophysiology. Too, Dr. Oh is the director of the Myasthenia Gravis Clinic at UAB.

Currently Dr. Oh serves on the Medical Advisory Board of the Myasthenia Gravis Foundation of America, Inc.

As a myasthenia gravis patient of Dr. Shin Oh, I have been very aware of Dr. Oh's distinguished background. I have been aware that he stays up to date through his own research, teaching, and patient care. I'm aware that he travels over the world presenting papers on MG and being on hand when his colleagues report their latest findings.

It was with this background in mind that I sat with Dr. Oh and asked him what he thinks is on the horizon in the future to help myasthenia gravis patients. I asked what he finds optimistic in the MG picture.

First of all, what does Dr. Oh find optimistic about the future in terms of facilitating research to produce new diagnostic and treatment tools for myasthenia gravis?

Dr. Oh is among medical experts who point very positively to the fact that myasthenia gravis actually is a disease that's relatively well understood. He notes MG is better understood than other autoimmune diseases such as multiple sclerosis, Guillain-Barré, and lupus. That understanding is important in researching MG—in uncovering information in the laboratory that can lead to breakthroughs in diagnosis and treatment. Dr. Oh said this understanding of MG holds the potential of being a big plus in the future in finding new approaches to deal not only with MG but also perhaps other autoimmune diseases that have similarities.

When Dr. Oh pointed out that medical science knows how MG works, he referred to an understanding about the antibody that is the culprit in causing MG. This is an abnormal antibody that has the power to alter normal body processes and thus makes MG known as an "altering disease." Because this antibody blocks or destroys the vital receptors for the neurotransmitter known as acetylcholine, the antibody quite appropriately is referred to as the "acetylcholine receptor antibody."

Dr. Oh explained that the understanding of this antibody translates to research potential that could help patients in the future: "We know there are many altering diseases. And we know that MG is one of these altering diseases. But, unlike many other altering diseases, what we know about MG is that we have an identifiable protein (the antibody) which can produce this disease. With this knowledge, researchers can produce experimental myasthenia gravis. Researchers can use the protein to trigger this disease in animals for research purposes. We don't have that knowledge with some of our other altering diseases. That's the reason why myasthenia gravis is much more ahead."

Secondly, as things stand today, what types of future new MG treatments does Dr. Oh view as being possible?

Dr. Oh was quick to pinpoint a big general area of hope—improvements in the field of immunology. He said this could come through new immunotherapy products tailored expressly to control myasthenia gravis. And he said a particularly big hope would be that a vaccine could be developed that would greatly reduce MG symptoms or even altogether cure MG patients of the disease. Dr. Oh is very much aware that one of his colleagues at UAB, immunologist/basic science researcher Dr. J. Edwin Blalock, is hard at work on a research project to develop a MG vaccine. As one who has treated MG patients for more than three decades,

Dr. Oh is very hopeful this research will bear fruit. "I really think this MG vaccine approach could be the way," said Dr. Oh. "And there's no question that I hope it happens."

10

RESEARCHING A
MYASTHENIA GRAVIS VACCINE

Dr. J. Edwin Blalock and his colleagues have developed a vaccine they hope ultimately can be used to greatly reduce or even cure symptoms of myasthenia gravis in many individuals.

This vaccine is not in the "preventive vaccine" category; that is, it is not designed to prevent individuals from getting myasthenia gravis, or MG. Instead, the vaccine is a therapeutic agent—designed to treat those who already have the disease.

"Ideally, we would like to see this vaccine be capable of producing a remission so strong it would in effect be a cure for MG. In other words, we would like to see the vaccine produce benefits that would protect an individual from MG symptoms permanently," said Dr. Blalock. "If the vaccine does not produce a cure, we would hope that the vaccine at least could enable many MG sufferers to enjoy major symptom relief that would last for years, perhaps even decades."

Dr. Blalock is conducting his MG vaccine research at the University of Alabama at Birmingham (UAB), where he holds the rank of professor in the Department of Physiology and Biophysics.

One of the reasons this vaccine research is so far along, said Dr. Blalock, is that myasthenia gravis is a well-understood disease in comparison to a number of other diseases that fall into the autoimmune diseases category. In speaking of autoimmune diseases, Dr. Blalock is referring to that category of diseases in which a patient's own immune system turns against the patient in some way. Dr. Blalock believes this MG vaccine research could have future potential in helping not only MG patients but also patients suffering from various other autoimmune diseases as well.

"Yes, it's rapidly evolving to a point where we think the procedure that we're using for this myasthenia gravis vaccine research can have applications to other autoimmune diseases," said Dr. Blalock.

Vaccine Research in Early Phases

Dr. Blalock has been conducting his MG vaccine research at the basic science level. The MG vaccine research he has conducted to date has been in the project's earliest phases—those phases related to developing the vaccine in the laboratory and the first use of the vaccine in animals. The vaccine has not yet been used with humans, and that cannot be done until extensive criteria have been met as set forth by the federal Food and Drug Administration (FDA).

In initial use of the vaccine in animals, Dr. Blalock and his colleagues found the vaccine to show effectiveness in rats and dogs.

The vaccine has been used in a laboratory rat model of MG—in rats that have myasthenia gravis which has been induced in a laboratory environment.

In using the vaccine in dogs, encouraging results have been achieved. In the case of the dogs used in the research, the dogs did not develop MG through a laboratory-induced process. Instead, the dogs developed MG naturally and spontaneously just as humans do. In ongoing studies, the use of this therapeutic vaccine has resulted in an 86 percent MG remission rate in the dogs that were treated.

The Vaccine Research Timetable

Even if this MG vaccine continues to show great promise, the vaccine must go through years of study before it can be made available for general human use.

How rapidly the research proceeds greatly depends on the availability of research funds and the speed of the research process. At this point, Dr. Blalock said his most optimistic projection would be a minimum of four to five years before the vaccine could be widely available to patients.

"To bring the vaccine to a point where it can be tested in humans, we must fulfill regulatory, toxicological, and manufacturing requirements set forth by the FDA," said Dr. Blalock. "This process is expensive and time-consuming. I estimate it will cost $3.5 million to fulfill the FDA's requirements."

This is the process the MG vaccine must go through before it can be tested on humans:

- **The first phase in the process is conducting the pre-clinical work prior to approaching FDA.** "This involves performing the initial research necessary to show there's a probability this MG vaccine approach is going to work in humans," said Dr. Blalock. "We have completed that phase."

- **The second phase is for the basic researcher—in this case, Dr. Blalock—to work toward obtaining from the Food and Drug Administration an all-important permit that's known as an "investigational new drug permit," or an IND.** To do this requires several steps and considerable time and money. The basic researcher first must meet with FDA representatives and explain what he wants to do. Whenever a researcher wants to make a new drug or vaccine, such as is the case here, the researcher has to provide the FDA with a "recipe" for the substance—that is, a precise formula for making the vaccine and specific manufacturing steps to be used in putting that formula together. The formula must be well designed, and it must show clear-cut chemistry. If the FDA agrees that the researcher can proceed, an approved manufacturer (a reputable laboratory) must be identified that will agree to contract with this project to produce the vaccine according to good manufacturing practices that meet FDA standards. "This is a major component of the expense and time involved in this type of process—the expense of hiring the laboratory to produce the material, and the time required for that laboratory to manufacture the material, in this case the material being the vaccine," said Dr. Blalock. As the process goes forward to manufacture a new agent such as a vaccine, the FDA has to have verification that several safeguards are being observed. For example, there must be proof that the vaccine is being made in a pure manner, there must be validation that nothing harmful is being introduced, and there must be evidence that the vaccine can be manufactured safely again and again with the same consistency. Then, once the vaccine has been produced according to these carefully controlled standards, toxicology studies must be conducted in two animal species. The FDA requires this in order to test the safety of the vaccine in animals before it is introduced to humans. Dr. Blalock explained: "What we would be doing here is taking this material that has been produced—the very same material that we plan to put into humans—and testing it in two animal species. These would be two animal species likely selected from among rat, mouse, dog, and monkey. And this animal testing, too, is a lengthy, expensive process."

- **The third phase is actually obtaining the investigational new drug permit, or IND.** After going through the process of having the vaccine manufactured and tested in animals, the basic researcher either is approved or disapproved by the FDA for the all-important permit.

- **The fourth phase is to go through the process to launch human trials—the testing of the new agent in humans.** If the basic researcher obtains the FDA nod of approval to receive the investigational new drug permit, or IND, the researcher can take his IND to the Institutional Review Board at his academic institution and request human trials on his new agent. It will be up to the review board to decide if the board agrees that what the IND-holder wants to do is sound and ethical. If the Institutional Review Board grants its approval, clinical trials can proceed. The clinical trials would entail monitoring by medical doctors who are clinicians treating patients with the disease that's the target of the new agent—in this case, patients who have myasthenia gravis. Sometimes a patient-based study will include more than one academic institution and perhaps several clinicians and their patients.

Dr. Ed Blalock and His Knowledge of the Immune System

Each time I review the status of Dr. Ed Blalock's MG vaccine research, my thoughts turn to what I know about the fascinating background of this researcher who probes into the mysteries of the immune system.

Before Ed Blalock set out to become a Ph.D. bench scientist whose work is in basic research, he was considering becoming a medical doctor who treats patients. However, while he was still a pre-medical undergraduate student at the University of Florida, he obtained a summer job with a professor in the field of medical microbiology/immunology. Young Ed got turned on to that field. He never looked back as he, too, pursued and obtained a Ph.D. in medical microbiology/immunology. "I just stumbled into something that I ended up loving," he said.

Early in his career as a researcher, Dr. Ed Blalock began attracting attention for his work in a field known as "psychoneuroimmunology." This has to do with how the mind influences the body, and, more specifically, with how the mind can influence the body relevant to health and disease. Dr. Blalock came up with a molecular and biochemical reason for how the brain and the immune system communicate. He reported on how the brain and the immune system actually have an overlapping chemical language. According to Dr. Blalock's research work, the same chemicals that run your brain can run your immune system and can also be used for the brain and the immune system to talk to one other.

Dr. Blalock attracted recognition, too, for his work on the theory that the immune system is really our sixth sense. He has theorized that the immune system makes us aware of certain conditions that we can't see, hear, taste, touch, or smell. For example, Dr. Blalock feels that the sensory function of the immune system acts as a sixth sense in giving us premonitions from time to time that we are about to get sick. He's referring to a subtle, non-specific warning a person can get from his body telling him in effect, "Something isn't quite right here, and sickness likely is not far away."

As Dr. Blalock moved forward with his research career, he used his knowledge base about the immune system as a significant part of his foundation to undertake new research in the design of drugs and vaccines. Some of his studies focused on a pattern in the genetic code that paves the way to design proteins, or peptides, that will interact with other proteins in a predetermined way. Dr. Blalock described his work about this pattern as one aspect related to what researchers call the "molecular recognition theory," a theory about how molecules interact. He said a number of researchers around the world are working on projects to broaden understanding of various aspects of this theory.

Dr. Ed Blalock also is very knowledgeable about how the immune system works in regard to recognition of shapes and contours. He has studied, researched, and made use of insight into how shapes and contours are among the driving forces in immune reactions. In fact, this relationship between immune reactions and shapes and contours has a significant connection to Dr. Blalock's MG vaccine research.

An Important Research Colleague

Some of the beginnings of Dr. Blalock's MG vaccine research date back to the mid-1980s. That point in time coincides with a transition in Dr. Blalock's career, with his taking on new research interests, and with his initiating collaboration with new research associates.

It was in 1986 when Dr. Blalock left the University of Texas Medical Branch in Galveston, where he had been for several years, and launched a new research career at UAB.

Not long after he arrived at UAB, Dr. Blalock joined forces with a Japanese physician who had an interest in autoimmune diseases. Together they put in place considerable groundwork for the myasthenia gravis vaccine project.

That Japanese physician was Dr. Shigeru Araga, a medical doctor who is a specialist in the field of neurology. Dr. Blalock credits Dr. Araga with important contributions to the early myasthenia gravis vaccine research at UAB.

"The way Dr. Araga and I connected was that, not long after I came to UAB, Dr. Araga contacted me out of the blue and asked about the possibility of his coming to the United States and working in my laboratory," said Dr. Blalock. "At the time Dr. Araga contacted me, he was with a medical school in Japan and was doing primarily clinical work with patients. He was at a point where he wanted to hone his research skills with the goal of furthering his academic career, and he wanted to come here to do it. So we made that happen. "

Dr. Blalock views the collaboration between himself and Dr. Araga as a win-win for both parties. "I believe in luck. And I think when Dr. Araga and I came together to work, that was a stroke of luck," said Dr. Blalock.

Dr. Araga already had an interest in how the nervous system controls the immune system. After he came to Birmingham, Alabama, to work with Dr. Blalock, he became very involved in Dr. Blalock's initial myasthenia gravis vaccine work. Dr. Blalock credited Dr. Araga as being the one who set up the laboratory rat model for MG.

"After Dr. Shigeru Araga set up the rat model for MG, he then tested the vaccine in the model; and it worked. Dr. Araga showed that the vaccine really was effective against that rat model of MG," said Dr. Blalock. "The other thing that we went on to show was that the way the vaccine worked was the way we thought it would work. That is, it worked through production of a beneficial antibody response."

Dr. Blalock said Dr. Araga's work was crucial to this project: "I wanted a good animal model; so that if what I was about to do worked, there would be a good likelihood it could translate into being something that would be of utility in humans. Dr. Shigeru Araga provided that model."

After working in research with Dr. Blalock at UAB for five years, Dr. Araga returned to Japan. Dr. Blalock said that today Dr. Araga is involved in academic medicine in Japan, where he has been conducting additional vaccine research closely related to the MG vaccine work. The vaccine research Dr. Araga is spearheading is exciting and, as with the MG vaccine, holds great promise in the area of autoimmune diseases, said Dr. Blalock. What Dr. Araga is doing, Dr. Blalock explained, is carrying out research on using the vaccination procedure approach to combat another autoimmune disease, Guillain-Barré syndrome.

Looking for a Well-Understood Autoimmune Disease

Even before he had pinpointed which disease he would target, Dr. Blalock had some ideas about developing a vaccine related to an autoimmune disease.

It was partly because scientists understood a great deal about myasthenia gravis that Dr. Blalock selected that particular autoimmune disease as the target for his vaccine work.

"I wanted to find an autoimmune disease that was sufficiently well understood; so if I came in and tried to change the course of that autoimmune disease, I would have a pretty good idea of what was going on," said Dr. Blalock. "As it turns out, myasthenia gravis fit the bill."

Dr. Blalock said that myasthenia gravis fit the bill both then and now for several reasons.

For one thing, scientists know what causes MG. They know that the cause is an abnormal antibody that is produced by the overactive immune system of the MG patient.

Secondly, scientists know what this abnormal antibody reacts with in the body to cause MG, and they know a precise location where the abnormal antibody interacts to do its damage.

Thirdly, there is knowledge as to how to cause myasthenia gravis in animals in a laboratory setting, and this makes it possible to conduct vital studies. "We can cause myasthenia gravis in experimental animals, including rabbits, mice, rats, etc.," said Dr. Blalock.

And fourth and very important, Dr. Blalock said the laboratory version of MG that is induced in animals is believed to be a match for MG in humans. He explained that this increases chances the same approaches scientists use to fight MG in laboratory animals ultimately will prove successful with patients.

"Unlike any other model for an autoimmune disease, the model for myasthenia gravis in rats or other species precisely mimics the disease in humans," said Dr. Blalock. "So the model for myasthenia gravis has virtually complete fidelity with regard to what you see in the human. Why that's important is that since we feel this model is truly virtually exactly like the human disease, then we have a lot more confidence that what we see in the animal can be translated into the human."

Understanding the AChR Antibody

A key element in scientists' understanding of myasthenia gravis is knowing about the abnormal antibody that causes the disease. That antibody is the "acetylcholine receptor antibody." It's also known by an abbreviated name, which is "AChR antibody."

In myasthenia gravis, what this antibody does is to interfere with the normal process by which voluntary muscles receive information from nerve impulses—information that's necessary for the muscles to contract effectively.

Since the MG patient has muscles that don't contract as they should, the affected muscles lose their strength and become very tired. The MG patient can have weak, tired muscles in various parts of the body—such as eyes, eyelids, arms, and legs. The MG also can weaken other voluntary muscles, including those related to smiling, talking, chewing, swallowing, and/or breathing. While one MG patient might have a MG condition that affects only the eyes and eyelids, another patient could have a condition that affects voluntary muscles scattered over the body.

As for how this muscle weakness is produced by the abnormal antibody activity in the MG patient's body, this is the process:

The abnormal antibodies multiply in the MG patient's body on an ongoing basis, as the patient's overactive immune system continues to produce them.

In causing their damage that results in muscle weakness, these antibodies wage an attack on vital receptors that are located on the muscle side of the neuromuscular junction. This is the area where the muscles and nerves come together to interact.

Actually, the name for this abnormal antibody relates to these vital receptors that are under attack. The antibody is called the acetylcholine receptor antibody, or AChR antibody, because it's taking aim on receptors that receive a vital substance called acetylcholine.

This acetylcholine substance normally is released by the nerve endings when the nerves are getting messages through to the muscles to contract. The acetylcholine thus has the important job of serving as a "neurotransmitter."

In the MG patient, damaging AChR antibodies are so active in destroying or blocking acetylcholine receptor sites that it's impossible for acetylcholine to do the job it needs to do—that is, help nerve impulses to get through to various muscles so the muscles will contract.

Dr. Blalock said a great deal is understood about the process in MG: "We know enough about MG to understand precisely where it is on the acetylcholine receptor that the abnormal antibody acts, and how it causes the problem."

But, he hastened to add, there is still much more to learn: "What we don't know yet, and what we hope medical science will come to understand in years to come, is what conditions exist in an individual's body to cause the immune system to start producing this abnormal AChR antibody in the first place."

A Therapeutic Vaccine

The goal of the MG vaccine developed by Dr. Blalock and his colleagues is to stop the production and/or action of the disease-causing acetylcholine receptor antibody, or AChR antibody.

"We would hope that this vaccine could bring about a permanent remission of MG, in effect a cure," said Dr. Blalock. "It is also possible that the vaccine might not bring about a permanent remission but instead a remission that lasts for years. And it could turn out that an individual who takes this vaccine might need to receive periodic 'booster' vaccinations to maintain the protection. That is the case with certain other vaccines that have been developed to address various health problems. All in all, I would hope that the MG vaccine will be capable of providing very long-lasting protection that will range from a minimum of several years, to decades, to perhaps a person's entire lifetime."

Dr. Blalock explained that some vaccines are designed to be preventive and some are designed to be therapeutic, and this MG vaccine is designed as a therapeutic vaccine. When a vaccine is preventive, or prophylactic, the vaccine is given before the fact—before someone gets the disease. When the vaccine is therapeutic, the vaccine is given after the fact—after someone has the disease.

As an example of a vaccine that is preventive, or prophylactic, Dr. Blalock pointed to the polio vaccine. An individual takes the polio vaccine to prevent getting polio.

As an example of a vaccine that is therapeutic, Dr. Blalock spoke of the rabies vaccine. An individual is given the rabies vaccine after he or she has been bitten by an animal that has rabies. The goal is to counteract the effects of the rabies activity already in the patient's body. "After a person is exposed to rabies, in all likelihood that person then has the rabies virus in his body. So you are starting the rabies vaccination after the fact. Thus the rabies vaccination in a pure sense is a therapeutic treatment as opposed to a preventive treatment."

As things stand now, individuals who are envisioned as the ones who will initially receive the MG vaccine are those who already have been diagnosed with MG, said Dr. Blalock. He said the goal would be to head off the abnormal antibodies—either by preventing the antibodies from being produced, or preventing the antibodies from performing their harmful actions.

Looking down the road, Dr. Blalock said if this vaccine proves to be effective as a therapeutic agent in MG patients, he can envision circumstances under which the vaccine's use eventually could be expanded even further. He said he can picture a time when this type of vaccine also could be used as a preventive agent, to prevent people from getting MG.

"However, before it would be practical to use such a vaccine to prevent MG, medical science would need to understand more about what triggers the abnormal antibody activity to be initiated in a MG patient. We would need to know this in order to predict who is likely to come down with MG, so we could identify who would need to receive the vaccine as a preventive measure," said Dr. Blalock. "For the time being, our first important goal now is to go through the process of testing this vaccine that we have developed; so we hopefully can get it approved to put into use as a therapeutic agent to help those patients who already have MG."

Anticipated Side Effects

At this point in his basic MG vaccine research, Dr. Blalock said he has no reason to suspect there will be serious side effects in humans who might ultimately take this vaccine. He added that research which still lies ahead will provide more information in this area.

"My feeling currently is that we can expect to see that same type side effects with this MG vaccine that we see in a number of other vaccines for various health conditions which already have been approved and are in use with individuals," said Dr. Blalock.

"These side effects could include perhaps a bit of inflammation at the site where the vaccine is administered and perhaps some myalgia, or muscle discomfort," he continued. "As with any vaccine, there is a risk there could be a small subpopulation of people who will suffer an allergic reaction. However, after vaccines have been subjected to the lengthy and rigorous testing and approval process, incidences of severe allergic reactions generally prove to be very few in number."

Implications for Other Autoimmune Diseases

Dr. Blalock is optimistic that the vaccine approach ultimately can be used to help patients with other autoimmune diseases in addition to myasthenia gravis.

What's needed to make that happen is to identify more "precise targets" in autoimmune diseases, said Dr. Blalock. If these targets can be identified—and Dr. Blalock thinks more and more will be—he said it will be easier to go after the targets with agents such as vaccines.

By targets Dr. Blalock means disease-controlling culprits, or villains. In part, he means if a vaccine is to be developed as a weapon against a particular disease, scientists must first identify the culprit responsible for fueling the activity of that particular disease. With MG, scientists know the AChR antibody is the target, or the culprit or villain.

Also, in order to use the vaccine approach to combat other autoimmune diseases, Dr. Blalock said more needs to be known about the precise places in the human body where these disease culprits do their damage. For example, he said in developing a vaccine aimed at MG it was important to know a couple of things about the culprit. First, it was important to know that an abnormal antibody is the culprit fueling the disease activity. Also, he said it was important to know that the place in the body where this antibody is doing its damage is on the muscle's acetylcholine receptors.

"What's happening today is that there's sort of a revolution going on in terms of researchers finding the precise places in the body that are being targeted in different diseases," said Dr. Blalock. "In different types of autoimmune diseases, we're getting better and better at identifying the target proteins that are causing the diseases. In addition to that, we're getting more and more instances where we know precisely within that target protein what sequence is being affected. So for many diseases, it's rapidly evolving to a point where the procedure that we're using for myasthenia gravis can be applicable to other autoimmune diseases. In principle, this approach we're using for MG should be effective against any autoimmune diseases where the precise targets are known."

In terms of research showing vaccine potential for more autoimmune disease battles beyond MG, Dr. Blalock pointed as an example to the ongoing work of his former colleague, Japanese neurologist Dr. Shigeru Araga.

"Since Dr. Araga returned to Japan, he has conducted laboratory vaccine research relevant to the autoimmune disease Guillain-Barré syndrome, which is a disorder in which the body's immune system attacks the peripheral nervous system," said Dr. Blalock. "It has been a couple of years since Dr. Araga set up a laboratory animal model for Guillain-Barré. What he has done is to demonstrate that the vaccination procedure is effective in an animal model of Guillain-Barré, just as it was effective in myasthenia gravis. I find this very encouraging. I view it as a fairly good indication that what we have here with the vaccine approach is something that has a good chance of helping MG patients, and in addition has broader implications for other autoimmune disease applications beyond myasthenia gravis."

Using MG Vaccine in Rats and Dogs

The first two animal species to receive the MG vaccine—the rat and the dog—received the vaccine under very different circumstances.

The rats were given the vaccine after they had been caused to have myasthenia gravis—after what is called a "rat model of MG" was created in the laboratory. In Dr. Blalock's vaccine research, creating that laboratory rat model of MG dates back to the 1980s and his collaboration with Japanese neurologist Dr. Shigeru Araga.

To induce the MG in the rats in the laboratory setting, the rats are injected with a purified version of acetylcholine receptors. These receptors are injected in a form to which Dr. Blalock referred as an "immunogenic form" to assure that the rats will get an immune response. "After a couple of injections, the animal—in this case, the rat—starts showing signs of myasthenia gravis," said Dr. Blalock. Then the rats are exposed to the vaccine.

By contrast, the dogs that have been given the vaccine actually have had spontaneous, naturally occurring MG, just as is the situation with a human who has MG. These dogs were pet dogs, whose owners wanted them to have the vaccine in hopes the vaccine would relieve the dogs' MG symptoms.

"As far as the dog studies are concerned, we got involved in that completely accidentally," said Dr. Blalock. "We got into it as a result of first performing an act of kindness for someone who had a dog that had myasthenia gravis. We actually were very surprised that the vaccine appeared to put this dog in remission. Then we subsequently used it on several more dogs."

Prior to receiving the vaccine, all these dogs had been treated with some of the same medications used to treat humans. The dogs had been treated with Mestinon® to improve muscle strength—by preventing the breakdown of acetylcholine and allowing more of it to accumulate. Also, the dogs had been treated with prednisone, designed to suppress the immune system and thus interfere with the body's production of abnormal acetylcholine receptor antibodies.

In treating the MG-stricken dogs with the vaccine, Dr. Blalock and his colleagues were able to bring about a MG remission in six out of the seven animals that completed the vaccination protocol. Dr. Blalock said vaccine treatment of these animals extended beyond being a research goal to also being a goal of helping the animals.

Dr. Blalock identified the six dogs that have responded positively to the vaccine as Buster the Boxer, Mollie the Collie, Pepper, Thunder the Great Pyrenees, Max the German Shepherd, and Poochie the Poodle.

These six animals responded so well that the vaccine seemed to virtually neutralize the abnormal AChR antibody activity, said Dr. Blalock. He said that after the dogs had gone through the vaccination protocols and were doing so much better, it was possible to discontinue the majority of their treatment with Mestinon® and prednisone.

There is a "great similarity" between canine and human MG, observed Dr. Blalock. Because of that, he said he finds it particularly encouraging that positive results came from treating the dogs with the MG vaccine. He said he views this experience as an encouraging factor in speculating whether a human MG vaccine trial might prove successful.

Theories Behind MG Vaccine

In conducting research on the MG vaccine, Dr. Ed Blalock has called on his extensive knowledge base and years of research experience relevant to the immune system and to approaches to drug design.

He said his work on this vaccine is the kind of project on which many a basic researcher thrives.

"One of the things most anyone in my field would like to do is be able to rationally design a drug or vaccine," said Dr. Blalock. "This is exciting. Because what you're doing is identifying a target enzyme or compound, and, in almost a predetermined way, attempting to design something that will go to that target and cause a change—some pharmacological change, for instance."

Dr. Blalock said that in attempting to design a vaccine that can ultimately be used to help someone who has an autoimmune disease such as MG, what the basic researcher really is doing is "looking for immunologic procedures to alter the course of a disease."

To do this, one of the basic premises Dr. Blalock worked with was his knowledge of a pattern in the genetic code that allows the researcher to design proteins, or peptides, that will interact with other proteins in a predetermined way.

"So you can say, 'I've got this big protein and it's got a site on it, and I want to design something that goes precisely to that site and binds there and causes some change,' " said Dr. Blalock.

In designing the vaccine, Dr. Blalock also relied heavily on his knowledge about shapes and contours as they apply to the immune system.

"The immune system works largely based on recognition of shapes," said Dr. Blalock. "Many interactions between molecules occur as a result of having complementary shapes, at least on the surface. This has application when we're designing a vaccine." He explained that researchers actually can work toward a goal of designing a vaccine that fits a site in the body where they want it to do its work. "What this process allows us to do is make something that we know in advance is going to have a shape complementary to the site that we want it to interact with. And that's an extremely powerful thing to be able to do."

All in all, in designing a vaccine to combat an autoimmune disease such as MG, Dr. Blalock said a goal is to restore some order to an immune system that somehow has gotten out of order.

"I suspect that in all people there's a balance between antibodies that are beneficial and those antibodies that are harmful and might cause autoimmune disease," said Dr. Blalock. "In a normal situation, these antibodies probably are kept in a balance, where this good one shuts down the bad one. And that's probably the way the immune system works. So I feel that one way of thinking about how these vaccines can work is that they can re-establish that normal balance, and get those autoimmune antibodies under control until they're essentially neutralized."

Doubt and Criticism—Part of the Process

Whenever a researcher is testing out a new theory, it's common for there to be many questioners, doubters, and critics, said Dr. Blalock.

He smiled and said there has been many a researcher who has discovered there was a fine line between being viewed as "infamous" because his research was doubted and later being viewed as "famous" because that same research proved to be valid.

"If you're doing science the way that it ought to be done, you are going to end up on somewhat of an island in a sense of becoming isolated," said Dr. Blalock. "If you're going about the process of trying to find out about something very fundamental, you're likely going to ask some question that nobody has ever asked before and as a consequence has never gotten an answer to before. So there you are, on the island. You just have to realize that you are going to be isolated, and you're going to be criticized. The more important the question you're addressing, the more criticism you're likely to get. Think about it. Virtually every major discovery comes about as a result of something that's unexpected. Most everything that is fundamental starts off as being unbelievable, a target for those who don't believe in it. I guess that's all part of the process of science."

Dr. Blalock described this critical process in relation to the MG vaccine work conducted by himself and his colleagues. He said while the MG vaccine work now is beginning to enjoy increasing support, the project has had to weather its share of criticism and doubt along the way.

"When we started this vaccine research years ago, it was considered to be heresy that anything would ever work this way," he said. "Although it's still not fully accepted, it's gaining in acceptance. And I think in the not too distant future we'll push it over the edge to even fuller acceptance."

Public Understanding of Basic Research

Having an opportunity to explain the process of basic research to the public is exhilarating to Dr. Blalock. He feels it important that people understand that most medical breakthroughs in diagnosis and treatment have their roots grounded in years of expensive, time-consuming research at the basic science level. He feels it important that the public realize the need for understanding and supporting vital basic research that occurs long before new approaches are tried on actual patients.

"In medically related research, there's sort of a set criteria by which we decide whether we should take a research project the next step and go into human trials," said Dr. Blalock. "Before we reach a point that we know we can do this, we have to establish some real probability that what we're doing is going to work in a human."

He explained there are many steps, over a period of years, by which researchers travel the road to reach that "real probability." This was Dr. Blalock's inside look at steps in that journey:

"Number one, we have this idea and we have a way that we think it works. So we go into the laboratory and we show that, yeah, actually this thing can do what we say it does in terms of how it's going to work.

"The next thing we do is we take an animal model of the disease that we want to try this in, and we try it in the animal to see whether it's going to work or not in the animal.

"In general, if it does not work in the animal, you don't go to the human. If it does work in the animal, then in that case you go through the processes necessary to try to get a permit through the FDA to test it in the human.

"So it's pretty straightforward. You do essentially what's required of you—what is required of you by the scientific and medical community, and what is required of you by the United States Food and Drug Administration. In so doing, you show that your research project—the drug, the vaccine, whatever—has shown efficacy in an animal model.

"That's what we have done with this myasthenia gravis vaccine. We've got a vaccine. We've got a system. Now we're ready to go forward with the vaccine manufacturing and with the toxicology studies in animals. We're ready to seek the IND permit from the Food and Drug Administration that we need to make this myasthenia vaccine available for human trials."

11

Opportunities for Autoimmune
Disease Research

As I look around at the many opportunities for autoimmune disease research, I am reaffirmed in my decision to set up a new foundation devoted to myasthenia gravis (MG) and other autoimmune diseases.

The MG vaccine research project directed by Dr. J. Edwin Blalock of the University of Alabama at Birmingham (UAB), which was outlined in the previous chapter, is an example of why I'm so optimistic.

More research initiatives in MG and autoimmune diseases are in the wings. I believe this new foundation can serve as a catalyst for even more.

As the foundation takes root and moves forward, we will be identifying research projects to encourage, to facilitate, and in many instances to finance. In so doing, I feel the foundation must be broad and inclusive in its perspective, rather than narrow and exclusive. We should not confine our interest to one type of research. Instead, we must explore many options on the tree's branches that we think could bear fruit.

Types of Research To Support

First of all, we must extend our support to bench researchers, to basic scientists, who have promising research projects in the autoimmune disease arena. If basic science projects are not supported, new knowledge will not be uncovered to combat these autoimmune diseases more effectively. Many well-trained, brilliant bench scientists are willing to invest a significant portion of their careers in basic research projects that could produce exciting autoimmune-related insights. To go forward, these researchers must have funding for their work. These are scientists who are trying to gain a better understanding of how autoimmune diseases play out their damaging activities in the body. Scientists are trying also to develop tools to reduce the severity of, or even eliminate, these damaging autoimmune activities.

In addition to supporting basic research, I think the new foundation I'm establishing must become involved in the support of promising clinical research. We must be supportive of research at the clinical level—research in which physicians and their patients participate—to test the effectiveness of new treatments on human beings.

At the beginning of this book, I mentioned still another type of research that I want the new foundation to address—epidemiological research that looks at the incidence and distribution of autoimmune diseases.

The Need for Epidemiological Research

I have absolutely no doubt that a great deal of epidemiological research related to myasthenia gravis and all autoimmune diseases needs to be accomplished in this nation. Since myasthenia gravis, or MG, is a particularly well-understood disease compared to some of its fellow autoimmune diseases, it's imperative that the new foundation focus first on supporting epidemiological research as it relates to MG. It's important because by learning more about MG we also open doors to learning more about many other autoimmune diseases as well.

As things stand now, so little is known to give us reliable, far-reaching data as to how many cases of MG probably exist in this nation and the geographical distribution of those cases. How many people in the United States have already-diagnosed cases of myasthenia gravis? And where do these people live? We have estimates and educated guesses. But I think that's about all we have at this point—estimates and educated guesses.

Obviously, even after we get a better handle on the number and the geographical spread of diagnosed MG patients, there still is another important side to that issue. This has to do with what many of us suspect is an unusually large number of *undiagnosed MG cases*. And I'm speaking of what I believe to be significantly more undiagnosed cases of MG than one would expect with a more "typical" disease—a disease with symptoms more familiar to the general physician community than those of MG. My personal opinion is that, by conducting extensive epidemiological research to take inventory of diagnosed MG cases, we will stimulate physician awareness and public awareness that in turn will help uncover many undiagnosed MG cases.

Why is it so important to have this epidemiological research? Why do we need to know how many MG patients there are, and where they live?

One reason we need to know is to be able to help these MG patients. If we can't pinpoint our MG patient population, we can't effectively extend to patients the services of MG support groups, discounted medication programs, participation in cutting-edge MG clinical research projects, and a number of other opportunities.

Another reason we need to know more epidemiology of MG is to aid researchers in learning more about MG and likely also learning more about other autoimmune diseases. If we're really going to confront this disease thoroughly from a research perspective, researchers need to know who has MG as it relates to sex, age, ethnic background, and family history of related diseases. They also need to have environmental profiles of where MG patients live. The more researchers know about the incidence and distribution of MG, the better are their chances of identifying patterns as to why these people are getting MG. Researchers can target groups of patients and look for answers to questions such as: Are pesticides related here? Are family histories related here? Is there a stress pattern here? For instance, I have a strong feeling (which I also have expressed elsewhere in this book) that future research will link significant MG occurrence to high levels of stress. In this book, three of the four patients who relate their stories are highly driven adult male professionals who had been exposed to high degrees of stress just before the onset of MG. Just in my home community of Birmingham, Alabama, several of the MG patients I know are driven professionals who experienced very high stress situations just prior to the onset of the disease.

Still another reason we need to know more about the incidence and distribution of MG has to do with funding for research. It's an indisputable fact that the diseases which tend to attract the most generous research support are those with the bigger incidence. We have generous funding in this nation to combat health problems such as heart disease and cancer partly because it has been obvious that there is a very high incidence of these health problems. With myasthenia gravis, I believe the disease indeed is a rare disease, in that I do believe its numbers are nowhere near those of health problems such as heart disease and cancer. However, I don't think the incidence is nearly as rare as it currently appears to be. I think more complete, accurate epidemiological studies will confirm that. And I want the new foundation to place a high priority on this epidemiological research.

From Basic Understandings to New Treatments

Despite the rare occurrence of MG and despite the fact that MG currently is a low-profile disease, many promising MG research projects already are under way.

These projects are widespread in terms of the institutions and researchers they involve. They are diverse in terms of the nature of the research projects themselves.

In this nation, MG-related research is in progress at medical and scientific components of premier institutions such as Johns Hopkins University, the University of Minnesota, the University of California at Davis (UC Davis), and the University of Alabama at Birmingham (UAB).

In other parts of the world, examples of institutions whose faculty members are researching MG include the University of Oxford, England; Weizmann Institute of Science, Israel; the University of Limburg, The Netherlands; and the University of British Columbia, Canada.

As one who is establishing a new foundation to address MG and other autoimmune diseases, I am enthused to see both the diversity and the quality of MG-related research. To me this says that a base for MG research already is in place. It also says that leaders of our new foundation will know where to look as a starting point for advisers, partners, collaborators, and also potential investigators the foundation could support.

As I look at the diversity of these MG-related research projects, I'm excited to see the different perspectives and approaches with which researchers are looking at MG.

One of the research arenas that encourages me most is the basic science work of some of the immunologists and other researchers who are learning more every day about how the immune system works. They are learning more about what is necessary to make the immune system work as it should. In doing so, they are learning more about what goes wrong to make the immune system cause damage to an individual in the form of an autoimmune disease. I'm speaking of autoimmune diseases such as MG, Guillain Barré syndrome, lupus, multiple sclerosis (MS), rheumatoid arthritis, type I diabetes, as well as many others. There are exciting research projects out there looking at cells, tissues, glands, organs, and other components of the immune system—the T cells, B cells, macrophages, thymus gland, spleen, lymph nodes, etc. In relation to diseases that are both autoimmune and neurological in nature (such as MG), I'm also excited to see some of the basic science work that focuses not only on the immune system but also in areas such as neurotransmission.

As a patient living my life with MG as part of the backdrop, and also as a physician, I can't express how optimistic I am about many of the treatment-related research projects that are in progress. Of course, some of the projects are aimed at developing altogether new treatments (such as Dr. Ed Blalock's MG vaccine research in Chapter 10). Also, there are other research projects—quite a number of others—that are looking more closely at the treatments we already are using. I applaud this research into the effectiveness and applicability of existing treatments. And I think we need more. We need more projects to look at the effectiveness and side effects of the steroid medication prednisone. We need more research into the use of medications such as Fosamax® to offer some bone-strengthening protection to patients who are taking prednisone. We need to encourage and expand projects that already are under way to look more closely at the use of the immunosuppressant medication CellCept® in the treatment of MG patients. I personally am excited about the potential of CellCept® to help bring an MG patient's malfunctioning immune system under control, without some of the side effects of the steroid prednisone and without the cancer-related risks of

Imuran® and cyclosporine.

One of my goals with this new foundation is for us to support research into a wide range of medications that can be used by MG patients to "put out the fire"—that is, to bring the acute stages of MG under control. From my personal experience as a MG patient and from my conversations with other MG patients, I believe a high-priority treatment goal with MG is to put out that fire. It is my feeling that the quicker you can get that fire put out corresponds to the quicker you can suppress the production of those damaging antibodies, the less damage you're going to sustain, and the sooner you'll be dealing with a disease that you are managing instead of allowing it free rein to manage you.

Segments of Myasthenia Gravis

Medical science already knows enough about myasthenia gravis to understand that there are a number of varieties of the disease and that these varieties affect people in different ways.

Often these categories are described as the "segments" of myasthenia gravis. There is promising research in this "MG segments" area.

These are some of the things we know about the segments of MG:

One type of "MG segment" has to do with the age at which MG is likely to strike and also how the age of onset tends to follow a gender-based pattern. Some researchers are looking not only at the age issue per se, but also at how symptoms can differ from one age group and/or gender group to another.

It's possible for a baby to be born with myasthenia gravis. That's pretty rare. But it does happen. A baby can acquire abnormal antibodies from a mother who has MG and be born with myasthenic symptoms. Quite often in those instances, the baby's symptoms will go away in a few weeks. It's also possible for a baby to be born with a myasthenic condition resulting from a defective gene that controls the proteins in the acetylcholine receptor or in the acetylcholinesterase enzyme.

Unfortunately, among the MG population as a whole, it's not rare for a child to have myasthenia gravis.

When a woman is stricken with MG, it's more likely for symptoms to first appear when she's a teenager or a young adult than when she's older. MG in women definitely is more likely to occur under age 40, and very often in the second or third decade of life (from age 10 to age 30).

For men, MG tends to strike at a later age than is typical for women. A more typical pattern with male MG patients is for them to begin feeling symptoms in their 50s or 60s. One area that some researchers want to study more is the abnormal antibody activity that's taking place in many of these middle-aged and senior citizen males who have MG. There are some theories that it's common for male MG patients to experience several types of abnormal antibody activity, and not just the basic abnormal antibody response against the acetylcholine receptors that's typical with MG.

Having said all of this, we also know that MG can occur in all ethnic groups, that it affects both genders, and that it can occur at any age. With an aging population, we can expect an increased MG incidence in both sexes.

Another type of "MG segment" has to do with the type of MG that one experiences.

You can have "ocular MG." This only affects the muscles of your eyes and/or eyelids, causing symptoms such as double vision and drooping eyelids.

Or you can have "systemic MG." A patient who has systemic MG can experience muscle-weakness symptoms in various parts of the body—including but not limited to muscles that control smiling, talking, walking, lifting, chewing, swallowing, and breathing. Some patients who have systemic MG have eye-related symptoms and some do not. *In fact, the symptoms are so varied and patients respond so differently to treatments that I am among those who wonder if all systemic MG patients really are suffering from the same disease process.*

We have just the beginnings of knowledge about the various MG segments. We need more. I personally feel that the expansion of epidemiological research will feed our knowledge about MG segments. As we gain more information about the incidence and distribution of MG cases, we'll gain more insight into the segments.

The Foundation's Roles

This new foundation that will focus on MG and other autoimmune diseases will not be set up to function as an island. I envision quite the contrary. In addition to fulfilling its roles as fundraiser and funder, this foundation will have as its missions the filling of roles as catalyst, conduit, and repository.

As a catalyst, the foundation will work toward encouraging and facilitating research among entities which might never have worked together previously, which indeed might never before have heard of one another. In addition to being a resource of funding, the foundation will be a resource for introducing compatible researchers to one another for potential collaboration.

As a conduit, the foundation will work toward becoming an organizational channel through which a wide spectrum of MG and autoimmune disease research can flow. In this area, I envision the foundation striving to bring about cooperation and collaboration among foundations with similar goals. The foundation should interact with other foundations that deal with similar diseases and encourage joint multi-foundation initiatives. As a part of this, I can even see various foundations referring research projects to one another and hopefully "cross-funding" some projects. By that I mean if another foundation has a research project that could potentially help with another autoimmune disease and also with MG, perhaps our foundation could help in that project's funding. Conversely, if our foundation runs across a project that has applicability to other diseases in addition to MG, perhaps other foundations could help us with funding the project. Also as a part of this conduit role, I envision our foundation having a constructive interaction with the National Institute of Neurological Disorders and Stroke (NINDS). This is the institute at the famed federally funded National Institutes of Health (NIH) complex in Bethesda, Maryland, that has direct responsibility for NIH research in the area of myasthenia gravis and several related diseases.

And, finally, as a repository, I envision the new foundation being a central clearinghouse for much of the high-profile research concerning myasthenia gravis and other related autoimmune diseases.

Times of Belt-Tightening and Scrutiny

To say the least, this foundation is being born into a challenging time in our nation's research-support history, a time that has no precedent.

For one thing, take the issue of ideas versus money. The ideas are plentiful. The money is scarce. On the one hand, never before in our history have there been so many promising research ideas to address the biomedical dilemmas that we face. Yet, on the other hand, the resources to fund those promising research ideas are drying up rather than expanding. It was in the 1960s and 1970s when I took my medical training and experienced the early years of my medical practice, first as a general practitioner and later as a specialist in obstetrics and gynecology. I saw firsthand those flush years when money was so plentiful for medical research. Today, those funds are more and more difficult to come by—at the federal level, state level, and private foundation level.

Then there's the issue of philanthropic scrutiny. The nation's philanthropic roots have been shocked by events and patterns of recent times. In the aftermath of the terrorist attacks of September 11, 2001, some high-profile charities have come under heated criticism. In addition, unrelated to the tragic events associated with terrorism, we have seen both church-related and secular recipients of charity shaken by questions and skepticism, in some instances associated with the taint of scandal and/ or the perception of misallocation of funds. The bottom line is that as a nation we now have a more suspicious philanthropic community. As far into the future as it's practical to speculate, recipients of both private philanthropy and government support likely will be under heightened scrutiny and have more rigid accountability requirements with which to comply.

For this new foundation that is emerging to tackle the mysteries of myasthenia gravis and related autoimmune diseases, I view the more stringent climate as an opportunity rather than a detriment.

Because of the shortage of research funds, we know we are needed.

And, because we know that we are starting out as a new entity with a clean slate, we have the opportunity to set up a well-administered, carefully monitored operation that can measure up to the current level of scrutiny. We will be aided by the high-quality members we select for our operating board, lay advisory board, and scientific advisory board.

The time is right for the birth of this foundation.

PART FOUR

MYASTHENIA GRAVIS PATIENTS
SHARE THEIR STORIES

THE STORY OF KELLEY HAUGHEY

I first met Kelley Haughey in the year 2000 in Chicago, Illinois, during the annual meeting of the Myasthenia Gravis Foundation of America, Inc. At the time, I was on this national foundation's board. I already knew of some of Kelley's successes as the executive director of the Garden State (New Jersey) Chapter of the MG Foundation—particularly her success with using walkathons as successful fundraisers. During the annual meeting session, Kelley and I shared ideas about securing funding for research to find a cure for MG.

I am so proud to have the story of Kelley Haughey's battle against myasthenia gravis included in this book. Compared to Kelley, I'm a newcomer to having MG, since Kelley was diagnosed with MG when she was 16 and has been battling it for more than a dozen years.

In her Myasthenia Gravis Foundation work, Kelley has become an outstanding leader in fostering the growth of the Garden State Chapter. She has involved her family and several of her friends in the chapter. She has put together a template fundraising model that can be used by other chapters. Kelley is extremely intelligent, very engaging, and has an outgoing personality that makes her instantly likeable. It's also very evident that she cares about those she helps, that she believes in her cause. She's able to walk into the offices of CEOs and convince them to support the battle against MG. Tenacious, persistent, and hard-working, Kelley has been able to increase her success every year with her MG fundraising.

Kelley is able to lead by example. That's unusual for someone her age. It's even more unusual considering that she has become a leader despite the fact she has MG—despite the fact that she has had a rough time with her MG. The thing that stands out uniquely to me about Kelley is this: She was so young when she got sick; and while some people that age would have been devastated and destroyed, she has done exactly the opposite. She has grown tremendously, both personally and professionally. Along the way, she has helped not only herself but many others as well.

The story of Kelley Haughey, as you will see on the following pages, is a phenomenal one.

RONALD E. HENDERSON, M.D.

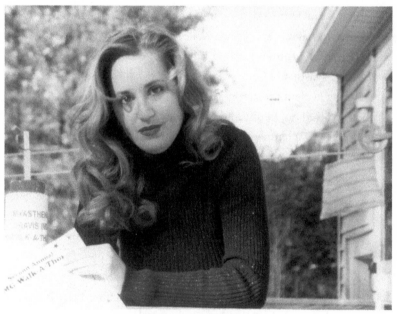

Kelley Haughey

12

An Early Jolt into Adulthood

By Kelley Haughey

When I look back at pictures taken of me as a child, I believe I had symptoms of myasthenia gravis, or MG, when I was as young as age four. In pictures of me at that age, I was not smiling; it was more like a growl. There's a little drooping of the eyelids in some of those pictures—another typical MG symptom.

During my early childhood there also was a fatigue factor. I was not a high-energy kid. I would just conk out and go to sleep very easily. That was a real contrast to my sister, Kathleen, four and a half years older than I. Kathleen was like Bugs Bunny, zooming around all the time.

Of course, those were things I didn't think much about until I was a teenager and had been diagnosed with myasthenia gravis. At age 16, when I was having trouble smiling, my eyelids drooping, feeling very weak, plus many other symptoms, my family and I thought, "Hey wait a minute. Let's look back at those pictures of Kelley at age four!"

Back when I was a little kid, no one really thought anything about it. Everyone thought I was cute—a four-year-old trying to smile and it coming out as a growl. The truth likely is that I *couldn't* smile because my facial muscles were weakened by MG.

Looking back and putting the pieces together, I think I went into remission after those first symptoms at age four. I think the symptoms stayed away until I was around 14. Then it took awhile for doctors to put all the symptoms together. I finally got a diagnosis when I was 16.

Sharing My Experience

As I relate this story in December 2001, I have just had my 29th birthday in November. Sometimes I feel as though I have lived many more years than 29.

I have a driving need to share my experience with others. I want to make the public aware of myasthenia gravis—to know what this chronic muscle-weakness disease is all about. I want to help other myasthenia gravis patients and their families, to help those who have not been diagnosed. I want to bring them hope and encouragement, and I want to bring them specific information.

It's easier now for me to bring the hope and encouragement. After periods of real crisis fighting myasthenia gravis, my life is going well. I have spent several years in college, earning both a bachelor's degree and a master's degree (business administration with a concentration in marketing). I have a job as an account executive with a public relations firm located not far from where I live in Wayne, New Jersey, about 15 miles outside New York City. Slowly but surely I'm working my way toward the independent life for which I have struggled so hard since I was diagnosed with myasthenia gravis.

Then there's my "other job"—that of executive director of the Garden State (New Jersey) Chapter of the Myasthenia Gravis Foundation of America. It just kind of evolved that I got that position. Several years ago, when I was still in college, I started doing some volunteer work in the MG Foundation office. One thing led to another, and two years ago I found myself in this top staff slot in the organization. As I have attended MG meetings around the nation, I've often found myself as the youngest person around in a leadership position. But, as I said, I feel like I've been grown a long time. I feel that I became an adult the day I was diagnosed with myasthenia gravis.

Knocked Down on the Soccer Field . . . and More

Being a teenager can be fun. It also can be challenging. Peer approval, being accepted, and being able to keep up with your classmates all are so important to a teen. As I entered high school I had no reason to suspect what lay ahead for me—that my challenges would far exceed being in the right group, attending the right party, excelling at academics and sports, and wearing the right dress and sporting the right hairstyle.

I could not envision that a rare and little-known muscle-weakness disease would grab hold of me. I could not envision I would endure a nightmare trying to find out what was wrong, be placed on life support three times the first year I was in treatment, and have to endure the emotional torment of classmates and even some teachers not understanding how this strange disease was affecting me.

The first symptoms I noticed during my teen years came during my freshman year in high school, while I was involved in sports activities.

When I was on the soccer field as a freshman, my knees started giving out and I would just fall down. I thought nothing of it then, especially since I felt no pain. Since I knew I was one of the smallest girls playing, I thought, "Oh, the big girls are just pushing me down."

When winter came, I had a little problem while I was skiing. I could make it down the hill; but at the end of the hill, where there are these little bumps, my knees started giving out.

Then there was this unexplained reduction in stamina that I felt as a member of the track team. In taking part in track at school, I always had done very well with distance. I ran the mile; that was my thing. I probably had it down to about a six-minute mile, which was good for high school. But by the end of my freshman year my six-minute mile had become my eight-minute mile. It was embarrassing to be on the track that extra time all by myself after everyone else had finished. I was devastated. I couldn't understand why my time was increasing.

In my sophomore year, things got worse with the sports.

I went to the first track meet but performed so badly I decided that was it; I dropped out. My coach and I had a very good relationship and I felt like I had disappointed him, but I tried to make it appear as though I had just lost interest.

In soccer I began falling all the time.

In trying to ski, I lost the strength to push myself up because my arms were getting weak.

Other symptoms appeared as well. I really liked to sew, but I didn't have the strength to put the thread through the needle. I had some double vision; it came, and then went away. I don't know why I didn't make a big deal of it, but I didn't.

Then one day at Christmastime I was trying to say "Jingle Bells" and I couldn't say it! Anything with a "J" or a "B" I couldn't enunciate correctly. Since my sister was studying nursing and was learning all that anatomy and physiology, I ran down the hallway to tell her. I was like, "I can't say 'Jingle Bells.' Listen to me!' " But then that speech thing, too, cleared up, at least for a while.

At school, my overall situation was deteriorating. Things I formerly had done I could no longer do. Like I always could beat the boys doing pull-ups in gym class; I always had been able to do that. But now I couldn't even get my fingers wrapped around the pole to pull myself up. Other things were happening. A teacher noticed that my eyelids were drooping, and he was concerned. When he asked me, "What's wrong?" I was like, "I don't know. I'm just really tired." By that spring there was at least one day a week when I wasn't able to go to school.

From One Doctor to Another

Like so many people who have myasthenia gravis, I experienced symptoms in various parts of my body that were so bizarre it didn't occur to me they were related. You don't think of a reason to connect these things all together as being caused by one health condition. I mean, *droopy eyelids* can be related to *weak knees?* So you tend to address your problems symptom by symptom, going from doctor to doctor. Most lay people and *many* doctors simply do not link together a patient having muscle weakness in various parts of the body and come up with a diagnosis of myasthenia gravis. Since myasthenia gravis is so rare and most doctors see so few cases, it's not uncommon for a doctor to miss it in making a diagnosis. To make it all that much more confusing, a patient's symptoms often tend to come and go. You can have terrible symptoms; but then, if you rest, the symptoms can just go away for a period of time. You might have symptoms and schedule an appointment with a doctor, but by the time you get to the doctor's office the symptoms aren't there anymore.

All too often these muscle-weakness symptoms sound so strange that (1) a doctor has no idea what's wrong with you, or (2) a doctor will wrongly diagnose what you have, often passing it off as something minor, or (3) a doctor will make it much worse for you by saying you're just imagining these symptoms, that it's all in your head.

I experienced all these scenarios. Since my parents were trying to help find out what was wrong with me, they, too, experienced this frustration.

One of the things I am trying to do through my work with the Myasthenia Gravis Foundation is to make people more aware of myasthenia gravis in order to help speed up a diagnosis for at least some people. That means the foundation's educational mission is aimed not only at the general public; it's also aimed at doctors.

In my case, I went from one doctor to another, trying to find out what was wrong with me symptom by symptom, trying to match the appropriate doctor to the appropriate symptom. My parents were there for me all the way. My parents believed I was telling them the truth about my symptoms even when some doctors misdiagnosed me, minimized what was wrong, or even said my symptoms didn't exist.

After the problems got so bad with my falling down during soccer, I went to an orthopedist and he said I had tendonitis.

When the double vision problems got worse, I told my mother and immediately she took me to an ophthalmologist. My mom was very concerned when she found out about those vision problems. One day I was sitting in the car with my mom, and I said to her, "You know what? I have double vision right now." She got really upset. Her reaction was like, "You have *double* vision?" She was thinking, "Does Kelley have a brain tumor or something? What's going on?" But by the time I got to the ophthalmologist's office, I wasn't having double vision anymore and the ophthalmologist didn't find anything wrong with me.

Also I was going to see my pediatrician about some of these different symptoms. At first when I told him about this muscle weakness, he said it was growing pains. But then as the weakness worsened and I was telling him about these problems in various parts of my body, the pediatrician took my parents aside and told them he thought I was just seeking attention, that this was all in my head. He questioned whether I was living a lifestyle that was a problem. He said maybe I was going out too much, maybe too much partying with my friends, maybe drinking, that kind of thing. He suggested that I see a psychiatrist. But my parents didn't do that. They believed me. They knew something physical was wrong with me and that I was getting worse.

Going Downhill Fast

By the spring of 1989 I was beginning to feel more and more isolated. I was so weak I was missing days from school and I didn't feel like going out with my friends. That's not how I had been in the past. I had friends. I liked to be loud, to clown around. I couldn't understand what was happening to me. I was thinking, "What the heck is going on here? I'm not really part of a group anymore."

I tried to stay upbeat and smile. But many times I was unable to smile, because I couldn't force the weak muscles in my face to make a smile. Many times when I tried to talk, it came out as slurred speech. The double vision was returning from time to time. I was asking all these questions: "Why can't I speak correctly? Why can't I smile? Why can't I see? Why am I so weak?"

Just getting dressed to go to school was a real challenge by the spring of my sophomore year. This was the late 1980s, and we had "big hair"—the poofy hairstyles with the teasing, the back-combing. Just to do my hair took a long time, because my arms were so weak. I would push a chair up close and prop my arms on the dresser to do my hair, and it would take forever. I would tell myself, "Okay, Kelley, get your hands up to get this hair done." It also would take me forever just to take a shower. Before I started having all these symptoms, I normally got out of bed in the mornings maybe 45 minutes prior to the start of the school day. Now I was getting up two to three hours before just to make it there on time.

There were times during this period that I would just lie on the couch downstairs and try to watch TV by burying one eye in a pillow so I could see straight, because of the double vision.

A Cup of Tea To Remember

One night at home when I was feeling really bad, my mom was trying to help me feel more comfortable and she made me a cup of hot tea. It was like, "Kelley, I know you're sick. Here you go. Drink this tea. Maybe it will make you feel better."

That's when another symptom hit me for the first time. My swallowing muscles shut down. I took a sip of tea and tried to swallow it, but I couldn't. It wouldn't go down.

Right away my parents took me to the hospital emergency room. I was so weak they had to help me inside. Well, we had to wait a long time before they took me back to the treatment area. We waited and waited, like two hours. During that time, I couldn't do anything but just sit; and I got rested. One of the things that can happen with myasthenia gravis is that if you rest sometimes the symptoms will get better on their own—at least temporarily.

By the time they took me back to the treatment area in the emergency room to see a doctor, I was so much better that I was showing very little symptoms. By then I could swallow. Although I had a touch of slurred speech and was showing some slight weakness, I was strong enough when I got reviewed by a neurologist that he thought I was fine.

The only thing they found that night was that in my blood test it showed I was a little low in potassium—which definitely was not my main problem. So they told my parents, "Oh, she's low in potassium. Give her some bananas and she'll be fine."

It was another miss in trying to find out what was wrong with me.

Finally—a Diagnosis

Although I didn't get a diagnosis that night in the emergency room, that event proved to be a turning point of sorts. After that experience, my parents were even more concerned. And since my mom was the one who actually was taking me to most of these doctors while my dad was at work, after the emergency room visit my mom was a woman on a mission! She was determined to find an answer.

My parents decided to take me to a local neurologist, Dr. Frank Gazzillo. He did a neurological exam. Although my symptoms were there the day I saw him, they weren't huge that day. Nevertheless, after examining me and listening to us tell what had been going on with me, he said, "Kelley, I think you have myasthenia gravis." He said he wanted to refer us to one of the medical centers for more input about the diagnosis and possible treatment.

Of course, my parents were very concerned when they heard I might have this rare muscle-weakness disease. My reaction? I was just glad to know *something*; I was so grateful to this doctor. I was like, "'Oh, thank you, thank you! You're the first doctor that's believed me." That to me was the *best*, rather than a doctor saying, "Kelley, it's all in your head." Also, this neurologist was referring us for further help, which I respected so much. I thought, "Oh, thank you for giving us some direction on where to go!"

Dr. Gazzillo suggested one of two medical centers. I guess you could say my parents chose both. We went for a first opinion to the University of Medicine and Dentistry of New Jersey—which usually is called UMDNJ—in Newark, New Jersey. And we went for a second opinion at Columbia-Presbyterian Medical Center in New York City. A neurologist at UMDNJ confirmed I had myasthenia gravis. At Columbia-Presbyterian, I got the Tensilon® test. They gave me the chemical Tensilon® to see if my symptoms got better, which they tend to do if you have myasthenia gravis. The test was positive. I had myasthenia gravis.

At that point I didn't know anything about this disease. But at least I knew that's what I had. I was just so glad to know. My thought was, "Okay, I have myasthenia gravis, okay."

My diagnosis came in April 1989.

Bring On the Treatments!

One of the first things the doctors discussed to treat the myasthenia gravis was to remove my thymus gland. They explained that this gland lay beneath my breastbone and played a role in my body's immunity. They said their goal would be to reduce my MG symptoms, although there was no guarantee of that. I knew they expected me to be in the hospital for several days, that they would have to put me to sleep, that they would have to split my breastbone (sternum). I also was aware that the surgery would leave me with a visible scar much like an open-heart-surgery scar, extending up my mid-chest to within several inches of my neck—high enough to show if I wore a sweater or blouse that had a scoop or square neckline.

But I was ready! I still was so focused on being happy to know what was wrong with me, and having people believe me and trying to help me. All this business about having surgery didn't really upset me; I don't know why. I actually felt more of a relief of like, "Okay, I'm going to get this operation that everyone's talking about, and I'm going to be fine." My only question to the doctor was, "Will I be able to play soccer in the fall?"

Reasons To Recall the Rough Times

In my current role as executive director of New Jersey's statewide chapter of the Myasthenia Gravis Foundation of America, I talk to many patients and their families. Often I share my experiences in order to help others. It is my hope that sharing my difficulties in getting diagnosed will help some people. That same goal is what motivates me to share some of the rough times and crises I experienced during the first year after I was diagnosed.

Some patients with myasthenia gravis don't experience nearly as many difficulties as I did. Some patients experience even more.

In reading this, I hope people will understand that for many patients myasthenia gravis is a very serious disease.

I also want newly diagnosed MG patients to be aware of possibilities. You could be among the more fortunate and have a relatively smooth path once you're diagnosed. However, you could experience some bumpy times during treatment, as I did. Just knowing these possibilities might help prepare you in case you're one of those who hits some rough bumps.

Another goal is a very positive one—to point out how well I'm doing now, to tell you that you can overcome even the rough times.

The First Round of Treatments

Looking back on when I started my treatments in 1989, in a sense I just don't think I really understood, or maybe I didn't want to grasp, what all was going on and what all was about to go on. Oh, I knew the facts about what was happening, just maybe not the possible implications. One thing I knew was that I had to undergo treatments in order to be better, and that's what I began focusing on.

The first treatments were medications. The medications didn't cause me any problems at the beginning. However, in my case, just taking the medications without other treatments didn't provide long-term relief either. When I first started on Mestinon® to help reduce the muscle weakness, at the beginning it made me feel like 100 percent! I started jumping up and down on my bed at home and saying, "Look what I can do!" My mom was my cheerleader and she was yelling, "Yeah!!" But the good effects of Mestinon® alone didn't last for very long. In June the doctors began giving me steroids, too. They were just trying to get me through the school year, so then they could add more treatments—plasmapheresis and the thymectomy.

Those additional treatments would help me. But the additional treatments also would bring complications I had to overcome.

In late June I had my first plasmapheresis treatment and suffered an allergic reaction to it. This is a plasma-exchange treatment in which they separate your plasma from the rest of your blood and replace it with fresh plasma or a substitute—a substitute such as a blood product called albumin. They were using the fresh plasma with me, and within a few seconds after they started my first treatment I suffered an allergic reaction to the plasma and went into a shock reaction. They switched to the albumin, and I tolerated it fine. Still, as a continuation of my allergic reaction to the plasma, I suffered a convulsion the next day.

I had only a few days to recover from the trauma of the plasmapheresis treatment before it was time to undergo the surgery to remove my thymus gland. I began confronting the reality I would have this long scar on my chest. I was 16, and a long scar on the chest is not exactly what a 16-year-old girl would welcome. On the eve of my thymectomy, I looked at my chest for one last time without the scar. I was thinking, "Well, this is going to change. So let me take a look at this like it is now." I did, and really I was fine with that. One thing that helped me deal with the prospect of having a scar and the overall idea of having a thymectomy was how bad I felt physically by the time the surgery date arrived. I was just so weak that my attitude was, "Let's do whatever we have to do. I'll just wear high-neck shirts and I'll put makeup over it and I'll deal with it that way." Another thing that helped me was that my goal was to be good and strong for my parents, because they were so strong for me. I didn't want them to see me upset. And then there was the positive attitude of the UMDNJ surgeon who did the procedure. My dad had researched possible surgeons for me and felt this surgeon was a good choice. He was. This surgeon had done a lot of thymectomies, and he was great with me. He did a good job with my surgery. Also, he was understanding in advance of the surgery. He told me that he had several daughters and that he would do his best to make my scar look beautiful. As it turned out, in the days and weeks after my surgery I would have many other things besides my new scar to think about. The first time I really looked at the scar would be after I was discharged from the hospital—several weeks after my surgery.

Many MG patients undergo a thymectomy and are out of the hospital and back home doing well within a few days after the operation. That was the goal with me. However, that did not happen. I was in the hospital almost two months. I had my surgery on July 5, 1989; and I was not discharged from the hospital until the end of August. In fact, the wedding of my sister, Kathleen, and my now-brother-in-law, Tony, got postponed due to my complications.

My first post-surgical complication was that my breathing tube became clogged. I experienced a breathing crisis, and they had to put me on a ventilator for a week. Part of the stress of being on the ventilator was just lying there with this tube down my throat and not being able to talk.

But that wasn't my only stress. An even bigger problem for me was *where* I was in the UMDNJ hospital when I was on this ventilator. You see, I wasn't in intensive care. I was in the hospital's big recovery room, for a whole week! The problem was that there were so many patients coming into that hospital. They were so overwhelmed and it was so overcrowded they didn't have enough places to put patients. So after my surgery when there was no room for me in the intensive care unit, that's when I had to spend a week on the ventilator in the recovery room. Now, this recovery room was just a big open room where you would just lie there, no TV to watch, nothing. And there was so much action coming in there that it was almost like an emergency room. It was disturbing. It was horrible! They brought in someone who had gotten shot, and he moaned the whole night and then he passed away. They brought in a little boy who had gotten hit by a garbage truck, and he eventually passed away. They brought in a pregnant woman who had gotten hit by a car, and they had to abort her baby. During that week there were times I really wanted to cry, but because I was on the ventilator I couldn't cry.

After I got out of the recovery room and was moved to the intensive care unit and was off the ventilator, there were more complications—problems swallowing, other things. I had to undergo more plasmapheresis with albumin. I had major problems getting my strength back. First I was moved onto a regular unit, then put back in intensive care, shifted around to other places, and finally discharged.

Returning to School

Amazing as it might seem considering my long hospitalization and all the complications, I still returned to school on time that fall. In September, the month after I got out of the hospital, I was sitting in the class-room with my peers, starting my junior year on schedule. Also, amazing as it might seem, two years later I completed my high school requirements and enrolled in college, on the same schedule as my peers.

Still, it was not a conventional road I took to completing high school. Although I returned to the high school classroom in the fall of 1989, I was in and out of the hospital for the next two years. Within the first six months of my return to the classroom, I was back in the hospital and on the ventilator twice. Once was Christmas Eve of 1989 because I got pneumonia; and the next time was three months later, in March 1990, because I was just generally going downhill.

In light of my hospitalizations and the up-and-down nature of my condition, I still think that my completing high school on time was kind of a feat in itself. There were times I didn't think I was going to be able to do it. Actually, I got pretty good grades, especially considering that I was sick so much. Many times it was so hard to focus on academics. Often instead of schoolwork I'll have to admit that my focus at the moment was things like, "What type of medication am I going to take?" and "Am I going to be able to get up out of the bed to go to the bathroom by myself?"

But there actually were times when school issues really helped me take my mind off my health issues. It's really strange now to look back on it. I recall that during one of those times when I was hospitalized and on the ventilator during my junior year, I would just lie there with my mind going over and over the amendments to the United States Constitution. I mean, there was only so much TV that I could watch, so I focused on those amendments. Now remember, I was a mentally alert patient on the ventilator. When you're a patient in that situation, it can get easy for those around you not to realize the difference in what you look like and what's really going on. I mean, you're unable to move your body and you're unable to talk and you're unable to express yourself; but your mind is so alive. Sometimes people can look at you in a way like they are tending to forget that your mind really is okay and alive. As I was lying there on the ventilator memorizing those constitutional amendments one by one, I just kept going over what the tutor had taught me. Pretty soon I could recall every single one of those amendments!

The Emotional Pain

For me, the physical difficulties of myasthenia gravis have been easier to deal with than the emotional pain. By emotional pain I mean the scrutiny and ignorance of others. I refer to some of the insensitive, sometimes nasty, things that people have said about me because they did not have awareness of myasthenia gravis and did not go to the trouble to find out about it and understand it. There were times when I thought perhaps I could see an end to some period of physical suffering, but I didn't know if or when all this emotional suffering would end.

I want to make it clear that this emotional pain was not dealt out by everyone. There have been *many* who have been understanding and supportive of me. Without those people I would not be where I am today. I'm referring to my family, many friends, some of the school officials and teachers, and some of the doctors. For example, there were school officials who were very lenient and understanding when I had to miss so much school—who really contributed to my being able to finish high school on time. There was a school nurse in high school, Nancy Przetak, who was wonderful. It's been more than 12 years now since she helped me so much, and I still talk with her. There was a period in high school after I was diagnosed when I would have to sit in Mrs. Przetak's office every day to eat my lunch, because I was having so many problems swallowing. This school nurse was great. She informed the teachers about my situation. She was so interested and wanted to know everything she could learn about MG!

Then there were those who brought the heartbreak.

The kids at school had seen me fall, slur my words, have droopy eyelids, not be able to smile, have no energy, and miss a lot of school. Then, after I was diagnosed and had to start taking a lot of steroid medication, I began to experience side effects of the medication. The side effects included fluid retention, weight gain, not looking anything like myself—being bigger and all puffy. My appearance was really altered. By the time I came back to school in the fall of 1989 following my thymectomy and weeks in the hospital, I already had gained 20 pounds on the steroids. Some of the teachers didn't even recognize me! Over the next six months, I would gain almost 20 *more* pounds.

Unfortunately, even though people had been told that I had this rare disease called myasthenia gravis, very few people really understood what myasthenia gravis was. There were those who disregarded any diagnosis they heard and instead came to their own conclusions.

I won't ever forget a day about a year after I was diagnosed when a girlfriend phoned me at home. It was a time when I had been very sick for weeks, including being on the ventilator again. I had been keeping up with my studies through home tutoring, but I was feeling better and getting ready to go back to school. When this phone call came in from my girlfriend, I was in my parents' bedroom and I took the phone call there. Actually, it's not especially important *where* I was. It's just that I remember *everything* about that phone call. As the phone conversation started, my girlfriend and I began talking about a lot of different things. The subject came up about a girl we knew in school who had been having an alcohol problem and had been in rehab. All of a sudden, just totally unexpected, my friend changed the subject with me and began to tell me all this stuff. She said, "Kelley, I want to tell you what people are saying about *you* at school because you're probably going to find out anyway." She said people at school were saying that I either had been in rehab for alcohol or drugs, or that I was pregnant, or that I had AIDS. I was flabbergasted! I just stood there in my parents' room with the phone in my hand and stared out the window. I was thinking, "So they're saying I'm not really sick with this thing called myasthenia gravis, but instead I'm having sex or pregnant or addicted or have AIDS? And how can I prove to them that I'm not?" I was like, "No!!!!"

This painful onslaught of misunderstanding and insensitivity did not end with the students. It extended to some of the teachers at school. There were some teachers who should not have reacted to me the way they did—some teachers who hurt me very badly. Teachers should know better. In my case, I was in high school and your high school years are tough years at best. When you're in high school, so many things depend on how you look, who you're with, etc. Teachers are aware of that. So when a high school student has a health problem, teachers should make an extra effort to educate themselves about that health problem and how it can affect the student. Also, teachers should learn about the treatments for that problem and how the treatments can affect that student.

There was a teacher who just didn't seem to understand about steroid medication and how it could affect patients—all about the fluid retention, the puffiness, the weight gain. The school nurse, Mrs. Przetak, had explained my situation to the teachers. But still this teacher came up to me and chastised me for my weight gain. She said, "Ohhh, Kelley, remember that old saying: 'A moment on the lips leads to a lifetime on the hips.' You had better stop all this eating." I mean it's not as though I wasn't already so sensitive and humiliated about how I looked. I just didn't know how to explain to this teacher that my overweight situation was not just a simple case of overeating. She should have known.

Then there was the day that a teacher yelled at me and hurt me so badly. And boy, did I react back to her, so strongly in fact that she kicked me out of her class. Immediately after she did that, I went straight to the school nurse, and apparently that teacher got in some trouble for what happened. But the damage already had been done with me. This occurred my first day back after one of my long absences, during which I had been on the ventilator again. At this particular time, I had missed my junior formal and lots of other things due to being sick. Here I was back in school almost 40 pounds heavier than a year ago. I was still so weak from this last period of illness that someone was having to help me carry my books from class to class, or my books were being placed in the classroom ahead of my arrival so I didn't have to carry them. But I was determined to get back into my normal routine. And it helped to know the school nurse, Mrs. Przetak, had briefed all the teachers on my situation. So here I go walking into this particular class. And there were some students who made it a point to greet me, asking, "Oh, Kelley, how are you doing?" I responded to the students. I was just so glad they were being nice to me. But the teacher had a nasty reaction to our having a bit of conversation at the beginning of class relevant to my return after being out sick. Instead of joining the kids in welcoming me back, she singled me out and yelled at me for talking, yelled at me in front of everybody!

Well, another side effect to this steroid medication I was taking is that sometimes it can make you a little jittery—actually, *really* jittery. Since I was self-conscious about how I looked, was feeling weak, and was really sensitive with my emotions, I just lost it with that teacher. As soon as she yelled out at me in front of the class, I went into a bit of "steroid rage" and yelled back at her; and she kicked me out. I just couldn't understand her reaction and I still don't. How could she do that to a student who had never before made any kind of ruckus in her class, and who was just returning after having been out of school for weeks including being on a ventilator three times in less than a year?

Finally, it really concerns me to report that some of my emotional pain was caused in a place it really should not have been, in a doctor's office. I say it *concerns* me because now that I'm an advocate for so many other myasthenia gravis patients, I wonder how much of that still goes on. If there's anyone in the world that you need to be able to talk with, and who needs to balance giving you the facts with also encouraging you, it's your doctor. About a year after my thymectomy, I was having a very low period and I was being really candid talking to my doctor. I was talking about how I felt battling this disease, wondering when or if I was going to be any better, and just wondering "Why?" about a lot of things. I was talking about how I felt battling this whole thing of ignorance, of people just not understanding—which really was even more stressful to me than the disease itself. That day when I went to the doctor was not a good day with my symptoms; I was slurring my speech a good bit. During the conversation, I began sobbing and just kept crying and asked the doctor, "Am I going to be better?" Instead of talking with me about treatment options and encouraging me, this doctor's message to me that day was dismal. Her basic message to me was, "Kelley, this is how it's going to be for you." Fortunately, my reaction was defiant and not defeatist. I thought, "You know what? You're wrong! It's *not* going to be like this for me. I am *not* going to be like this!"

A Supportive Family—Something to Treasure

When you have a chronic disease, it's a real treasure to have your family stick by you.

My family has been there for me. No matter how difficult things have been for me at times in my battle against myasthenia gravis, my mother and father (Georgine and Kevin) and my sister and brother-in-law (Kathleen and Tony) always have been there to do whatever was needed.

In the months leading up to my MG diagnosis, my family believed me when I said I was having these strange come-and-go symptoms of weakness in various parts of my body. They believed me even when doctors were doubting my story.

After I started treatments my family was there in so, so many ways.

When money became an issue to pay for some of my treatments, my family was there. My parents pushed for insurance coverage for my treatments, and they paid many out-of-pocket expenses not covered by insurance.

And, as I escalated my work with the Myasthenia Gravis Foundation's Garden State Chapter, my family helped me. In fact, I moved the chapter's office into my parents' home!

I have felt a close bond with my family all my life. My father is a tax accountant for American Home Products. My mom has been a stay-at-home mom. My parents always have really focused on my older sister, Kathleen, and me. I remember really good times from my childhood. Like the Sunday morning family thing. Every Sunday was special. My mother and father and Kathleen and I would have Sunday breakfast together, and then together we would go to services at the Roman Catholic church where we were members.

That's the way it was—the four of us, really close. After Kathleen met and became engaged to Tony Wade, to me it was not like I was getting a brother-in-law but instead like Tony was my new brother. After Tony came, our family became the five of us instead of four, all still really close.

When I got sick with myasthenia gravis, it wasn't just *my* illness; it was a *family* illness. That's how it should be with a chronic disease; because when one member of the family develops a chronic health problem, that person needs the support of the entire family.

My battle against myasthenia gravis has been a battle for my entire family.

When I was in the hospital, there was always someone there with me. My mother would spend the nights with me in the hospital and stay a lot during the day. My father would come after work. My sister, who was studying to become a nurse at the time, would come between her classes and give my parents a rest. Tony started helping even before he and Kathleen married, and he continued to help after they married. He would help with cleaning my parents' house, with making dinners and all that. He was the person saying to me things like, "What do you need at the hospital? Do you need fresh pajamas? Anything else I can get for you?"

Any hospital patient in the kind of situation I was in needs someone to serve as an advocate. My family really came into the picture on that. When I was lying there on a ventilator, I couldn't fight for myself; I needed somebody else to fight those battles for me. I needed someone to speak for me because I couldn't speak. Even when I wasn't on a ventilator, I often was lying there so weak that I needed someone to speak up about things such as if the nurses were late with my medicines. That kind of thing happens in a hospital. Often it's not really the fault of the nurses and the other people taking care of you, because so many times they just have too many patients to take care of with too few hospital staff members. So you really do need your family as your advocates, to speak up for you.

When you're going through a particularly difficult health crisis—something you just don't know how you're going to make it through—having family members to support you means everything in the world. There were *many* rough times when I don't know what I would have done without my family there. But one time that especially stands out in my mind is when I was in the hospital in March 1990. It was almost a year after I was diagnosed. I had been going downhill and they were putting me on the ventilator again, for the third time. Since I was having so much trouble swallowing, they decided not to insert the ventilator breathing tube by going through my mouth, which is the usual way, but instead to put it through my nose—to intubate me through my nose. What took place after they made that decision would create the absolute worst memory I have of any of my treatments—worse than anything with my thymectomy, the plasmapheresis, anything! As the doctor started inserting this tubing down through my nose, I was alert and aware of everything going on. I also was already in great distress—couldn't breathe, couldn't swallow, and was very, very weak. Getting that tube in place turned out to be the most painful thing I have ever experienced in my life. It took three nurses to hold me down! On the first try the doctor didn't get it in the right passageway, and they had to pull it up and do it again. It was awful. For a month after that I had scabs coming up from all that scraping all the way down. Afterward I was in so much pain and had such a headache they had to give me morphine. My blood pressure went up so high they were afraid I was going to have a stroke, and they had to put me on blood pressure medication. Suffice it to say that I remember this ordeal like it was yesterday. I also remember that my family was there to help me get through it.

My family also has been incredible when it has come to helping me evaluate which treatments I should take, conducting research to decide which health professionals should perform these treatments, and finding means to pay for these treatments. One thing my parents have done for me with my healthcare that I especially appreciate is that they always have respected my role as being the patient. My parents did not make the decisions for me about which doctors to see. They looked into options; they found out about backgrounds of various medical and surgical teams and whether certain people were qualified. But when it came down to a final decision, they put the question to me of, "Kelley, who do *you* feel comfortable with? We know this team is good; we know the other team is equally good. What do *you* think?"

As is true with any patient with a chronic disease, you have to find the treatments that work best for you. No one treatment regimen fits everyone. What works for one person might not work for another. For me, one of the treatment approaches I feel really helped was the use of an intravenous drug treatment called IVIg—or intravenous immunoglobulin, often called by such names as immune globulin or gamma globulin. It didn't prove to be a quick fix for me, but it was something that stabilized me. I've never been on life support since I took the IVIg, and I credit that treatment with being one of the reasons for my improved condition. I credit my parents with helping me to obtain it and pay for it. When I started on this treatment in April 1990, it was still considered experimental in many circles. It was a new type of treatment they were just beginning to use on myasthenics. That meant if you were a myasthenic at that time you might not even find out this treatment existed. I think it was due to being in the right place at the right time that my mom and I learned about it. I was a patient in the hospital intensive care unit. My mom was there with me. Some neurologists were there at the hospital for a conference and said, "Hey, we've got a myasthenic in ICU. Let's take a look at her." When the neurologists came by to visit, they told my mom about IVIg and gave her some information on it. She kept the information, pursued it, and said, "Let's look into this!" Another thing about a new medicine like this is that it can be very expensive. This IVIg indeed was very expensive. When I started taking IVIg, the cost for a month's treatment could range from $18,000 to $22,000. Also, when you're dealing with an expensive and costly product that's new, with little data out there to say this is going to work, it can be a battle to get the insurance company to pay. I thank my parents for pushing the doctor to write letters to the insurance company, to get the IVIg for me. Without my parents' help I never would have gotten that IVIg.

Without my family's support, I wouldn't have gotten a lot of things I have needed since myasthenia gravis came into my life. Without my family's support, I don't think I would be living the full and productive life that I enjoy living today.

Getting to Where I Am Today

I think for many MG patients the first few years after diagnosis are the toughest. I know that has been my experience. It has been almost 13 years since I was diagnosed, and all in all I'm doing well. My life is full—with my full-time public relations job, heading my state's chapter of the Myasthenia Gravis Foundation, going out with friends, taking some personal trips and some trips for the foundation.

Now, don't get me wrong; my health picture is not perfect. I still have myasthenia gravis. It's just that my MG is more under control than it was years ago. It's being managed, and I'm not going through crisis after crisis. The symptoms are less severe. Oh, there are days when I feel less energetic than others. There are times when my eyelids droop, when my facial muscles are so weak I can't smile, and when I slur my speech. And there still are times when these symptoms depress me a bit. But the medications do a pretty good job of keeping them under control.

I take considerably less medication than I did years ago. In 1990, when I went into my first IVIg treatments, I was on high dosages of oral medications. I was taking 120 milligrams of Mestinon® about every two to two and a half hours, and I was taking 100 milligrams of the steroid medication prednisone every day. Today I take 60 milligrams of Mestinon® as needed, the exact amount depending on what's going on with me that day, including the level of stress I'm under. Some days I take the Mestinon® only once or twice; on a real stressful day I take it maybe four or five times. I am no longer taking the steroids, the prednisone. After I had taken prednisone for eight years, the doctors were able to taper me off gradually until I was taking none at all. That's how you have to do when reducing steroids; it has to be a gradual reduction in your dosage that's monitored by your doctor. (One good thing about getting off the steroids is that my weight is back under control; I'm back to the 105 pounds I feel comfortable with for my height of 5 feet, 2 ½ inches.) I still credit the IVIg treatments with helping to stabilize me and keep me stabilized. During this past year—the year 2001—I took two treatments of the IVIg, one in March and one in June. When I take IVIg now, it's with a much lower dosage of the medication. Now I take 30-gram treatments, as compared to 105-gram treatments back in 1990.

While I know the medical treatments I have received no doubt have played a big role in my being able to live an active life today, I don't think they're the only reason I'm doing well. In my opinion, attitude also has played a tremendous role.

Again, my family helped me as I formed my attitudes about my illness. My family's faith really helped strengthened my own faith in my future. There were times when I think my doctors went overboard in encouraging me to accept too many limitations because of my MG, while my parents were encouraging me *not* to accept too many limitations. I decided I would not allow myasthenia gravis to rule my life.

I've had to have a strong religious faith about all this. I mean, when you get something like MG, you tend to ask the question over and over, "Why me?" But eventually for me I just knew that God did not make me have this disease. I also knew that I had to have the strength to move on.

In making my decision not to let MG rule my life, I had to develop a determination to help manage my own illness in a way to keep from getting into deep trouble again. I would look back at those days on life support and I would tell myself I *had* to prevent that from ever happening again. Then I would ask myself, "So what can I do to help prevent that from happening again?" That's what drives me now when I manage my medications, when I decide it's time for an IVIg treatment, and when I'm really tired and I carve out time in a busy day to take a nap.

To be as active as I am and to mingle with the public as much as I do, I had to realize that I was doing some things the *wrong way;* and I had to make necessary corrections. One of those "corrections" is that I had to become more open with people about my having MG, so that I could live an active life without fear that I was going to embarrass myself in some way. I finally had to come to the conclusion that I refused to be ashamed anymore. This has been a real contrast to the earlier years of my disease, when I tried to hide from many people the fact that I had myasthenia gravis. I didn't like having the tag or label of being sick. I was afraid that people were going to judge me because I had a chronic illness. Then, one day during my sophomore year of college, I suffered a humiliating experience that made me realize I was going to encounter more problems by *not* informing those around me that I had MG than by informing them. This humiliating collegiate experience took place in the classroom, in a management information systems class. I had told my teacher in this class that I had MG; in fact, I had explained my MG to all my college teachers. I had let the teachers know that due to MG I might be absent some from class and that I might have MG symptoms while in class. However, I had elected not to inform my classmates about the MG, because of that fear I had of being labeled chronically ill. Well, in this management information systems class we were required to make a speech. I felt some anxiety about this, because I was afraid when it came time to give the speech I would slur my words and be embarrassed. When the day came for me to give the speech, I indeed was experiencing some MG-type weakness and I asked the professor if I could delay my speech until the next class period. Even though this professor knew I had MG, he took a real hard line. He accused me of being unprepared. I told him, "I'm not unprepared. It's just that I can't speak *today.* Please, let me just do it the next class." He told me, "Kelley, if you don't give the speech today, you get a zero." So, not wanting to take that zero, I stood and made my way to the podium in front of the class to give the speech. As I walked up, I felt weak and anxious. I told myself, "Oh, Kelley, you *can't* slur; you've *got* to cover up this MG." Well, the worst happened. When I tried to say the very first word of my speech, I physically could not do it. I couldn't speak. The professor made an example of me. He said, "If you come to class unprepared like Kelley, you'll get a zero!" I just walked off the podium and out of the classroom, totally humiliated. I fully believe that I would not have been as terrified that day if I had alerted not just the teacher but also the students in the class, if everyone in the classroom had known about my MG. So from then on, I not only told all my teachers about my MG; I also told my classmates. In every situation where I thought it mattered, I told my peers, "Look, I have myasthenia gravis. This is what it is. These are the symptoms. This is what can happen." Still, it took time for me to overcome that experience. My humiliation in that classroom that day began for me a real fear of speaking in public. I just didn't think I could do it anymore. Then, after I decided to go on to graduate school, I had no choice. We were required to make speeches in all our graduate classes. It took some doing for me. The first time I tried to speak in front of a graduate class I was so scared I literally passed out! The next time, I managed to get through my speech; but it was not a very good speech. Then gradually I started improving. And it helped so much that I was open about my MG with everyone in the audience. The students were so cool about it. By the time I completed my master's my classmates were really rooting for me, like, "Great job, Kelley!" It was good that I was pushed into overcoming that terrible fear of speaking. While speaking still is not my favorite thing, I do a lot of it in my role as executive director of an MG chapter!

No doubt one of the hardest things for me emotionally in recent years has been learning patience—maintaining patience during my ongoing quest to attain my full independence as an adult. I'm doing better with that, but it's a continuing struggle.

If you're an independent-thinking teenager—and I was one of those—no matter how much you love your family, you look forward to leaving home and going off on your own to college, and, after that, getting a job and a place of your own to live. Just doing the independent thing.

While I know that things have gone well for me in recent years despite MG, I also am aware that MG has gotten in the way of my independent path. I've had to learn to go forward in spite of that. When I completed high school requirements and was ready for college, I still was so symptomatic with MG that I simply was not well enough to go away to college. So I stayed home and enrolled in William Paterson University in my hometown. That's where I earned both my bachelor's and master's degrees. I think I helped fuel my own motivation during my college years because I set some high standards for myself and got pretty close to them. I made it a goal to get straight A's. Although I made a couple of B's that bothered me, I did mostly make A's.

After college, MG still was getting in the way of my following an independent path. Initially when I was out there looking for a job, I still had a lot more active MG symptoms than I'm having today. That hampered my getting the kind of job I sought with the kind of health insurance coverage that I needed. The work I had begun and continued to expand with the MG Foundation was important to me. However, even after I stepped from volunteer role into staff role in the foundation and started getting paid, I wasn't making much money. I wanted then what I still want today (and what I *have* today); I wanted to keep doing MG work and also hold a *real* job. I wanted the things that young women in their 20s typically want. I wanted to have my own money, I wanted to buy my own car, and I wanted to find my own place to live. My friends in my age group had moved on to do these independent things, while I was still living at home with my parents and my only job was a modestly paying one related to my chronic disease. Although my friends weren't judging me in this regard, to me I felt that people were defined by, "What do you do? Where do you work?" I felt held back. Today I'm glad to report that things are much better for me in this area. They're better partly because I've made some progress in attaining segments of my independence, and they're better partly because my attitude has improved about accepting the fact I still have segments of my independence I have not yet attained. About a year and a half ago I was able to get that job I wanted, with good group insurance. Last month I bought my first car. I'm working toward getting my own place. In regard to attitude improvement about all this, I've come to the point that I really know how lucky I am. I look at myself like, "It's okay that you're still living at home, Kelley. You're going to get your own place; you're going to get there. But for now, you're lucky you can stay home and that you have the support of a family who can and does help you." Actually, I'm lucky to have the support of a family who not only has reached out to help *me*, but also to help me in my efforts through the MG Foundation to help *many others*—other myasthenia gravis patients and their families.

Working with the MG Foundation

It was at the suggestion of my father that I began doing volunteer work with the Garden State Chapter of the Myasthenia Gravis Foundation of America, Inc. Just as I could have no idea I would develop full-blown myasthenia gravis as a teenager, I also could not predict that I would become so bonded to working to help other myasthenia gravis patients and their families.

At the time I first started doing volunteer work, I was just completing my bachelor's degree requirements in college and had a little time before I started my master's work. I really wanted to get involved in something in addition to school. Prior to getting MG, I had done sports—soccer, skiing and track. Now I needed to find something else. My dad said, "Kelley, why don't you volunteer to help out with the MG Foundation?" The office of the MG Foundation's Garden State Chapter was in a town about 20 minutes from my home.

Now, looking back over how deeply I have become involved in MG work, I recall my dad's first suggestion and smile. I think, "Boy! Famous last words those were!"

When I started out with the Garden State MG Chapter, I was 22 years old, the youngest volunteer coming in to help the chapter. There were some volunteers who had been giving time there for years. At first, I just helped with doing some photocopying; I don't even think I was allowed to answer the phones. And you can't blame them. I mean, what did I know about running an office?

Next I moved on to a bigger task at the chapter, that of helping them with their quarterly newsletter. Just getting all those newsletters out in the mail was a job within itself.

Then I had an experience that made me want to do something really major for the Myasthenia Gravis Foundation's Garden State Chapter, in terms of making people more aware of what myasthenia gravis is all about. What happened was that I had another spell of illness. It was a really bad sinus infection, with high fever. That made my MG symptoms worse. I was hospitalized—in intensive care for a week. The doctors and nurses were great, and they worked with me to keep me off the ventilator rather than just throwing me immediately on life support. However, in the course of this I was having to inform some of these doctors and nurses about MG. They were asking *me* to tell *them*. I thought, "There's just so little awareness of MG. I have to do something to elevate the awareness."

From then on that became my thing—MG awareness, MG awareness, MG awareness!

So I got the idea of holding a walkathon—a walkathon that could raise some money and also spread awareness about MG. I went to the people at the Garden State Chapter and said, "Look, I want to do this walkathon." They were like, "Okay." The only thing was they had no money for it, no budget. The only help they could give me was some chapter letterhead. But that was fine; that was understandable. Really, I wasn't even asking them for a budget.

I had never done fundraising in my life. I asked some of my friends to help me with the work to put the walkathon together. I used $100 of my own money to pay for basic things we needed. We held our first walkathon in 1998. We cleared $11,000 with that walkathon. And we spread the word about myasthenia gravis.

The next year, we held another walkathon and we cleared $24,000. Included in that year's profit was a single $10,000 donation from an elderly woman who read my story in the local newspaper.

We continue to have our walkathon each year, and we continue to do well.

The walkathon has attracted the interest of some other chapters of the Myasthenia Gravis Foundation. I've also appeared before some board members of the national foundation to explain the walkathon. It is my dream that one day we will hold a national walkathon for myasthenia gravis—a national walkathon event made up of local walkathons for MG held around the nation on the same day.

I think the success of our walkathon played heavily into my becoming executive director of the Garden State Chapter. There were those on the chapter's board who were so pleased with the success of the walkathon that when our executive director stepped down they asked me to take over the position. I think once I had proved myself, that's when people said, "Okay, we'll let Kelley run the chapter."

My reaction was that I really didn't want to take on that big of a role. By this time I was deep into my studies toward my master's degree, and I felt I needed to devote my energy to finding a "real job." I had started with the MG Foundation's Garden State Chapter as a volunteer, and I viewed that as my role. But, even though I didn't want to take on the executive director position, there was a need. And I did take it over. I felt if I didn't take it over the Garden State Chapter might not continue to be there. I felt I had to accept the leadership position. I became executive director in 1999.

The chapter had some real needs, some real gaps. Over a period of several years, some board members who had done considerable volunteer work had passed away. And no longer were there people there to fill roles such as program director, health fair program director, and accounting manager.

To help with the tremendous amount of work that needed to be done, I recruited some of my friends and members of my family as board members for the chapter.

A couple of my friends, Deniele DeBoer and Diane McDermott, became board members even before I took over as executive director. Two more friends, Kelly Good and Dara Zumbo, came on the board after I accepted the executive director job. These four friends already had helped me out so much with the walkathon. I told them, "Come on and be a board member, and you can put this on your resumé and get credit." Today I have them to help me out with the health fairs where we inform the public about MG. And they are the ones who figure out the programming for our general meetings four times a year—events for which we get speakers.

My family members who became board members are my mom, my dad, and my sister. They have helped me more than I can say with the work of the board.

My mom and dad also went the extra mile in opening their home to the Garden State Chapter of the Myasthenia Gravis Foundation of America. From the start, when I was offered the post of executive director, I knew I planned to get a full-time job in addition to the MG job. I knew that to balance all this I had to make things as streamlined as possible, so I could make the most of evening and weekend hours. So I got this idea. I said, "Mom, Dad, can I bring the office of the Garden State Chapter home with me and let it occupy a room at the house?" There was no question in their minds. They said, "Yes." So the chapter office moved into our home.

Nine months after I accepted the executive director job, I received my master's degree. Three months after that I landed that "real job" I had been seeking, the public relations position. At this point, I informed the board of the Garden State Chapter and told them that if they wanted to give the executive director post to someone else they could. No one came forward for the position. So I stayed on.

I continue to love what I'm doing with my MG work. In doing this, I know it has been therapeutic for me. I get so much satisfaction when I can help someone with something that I can understand all too well.

In my role as executive director, I get phone calls from people who are newly diagnosed with myasthenia gravis. They need information badly, and I can get that information to them. I've been where they are now. I feel it's my obligation to help these people.

I have goals in reaching out to help these people—those who have been diagnosed and those who are not yet diagnosed. If we at the Garden State Chapter can take steps that help prevent people with MG from going months without a correct diagnosis, help prevent them from going on life support, and help prevent them from being humiliated because of the ignorance of others, then these are good things and we have to do them. I really have to say that dealing with the ignorance of others, the getting made fun of because you look different or because you can't smile, is harder than any thymectomy, any plasmapheresis, any type of medication you can be on. It's the worst pain that you can feel. And when you feel alone, that's worse. What hope do you have? I don't want people to go through that. I want them to know they are not alone.

As far as MG research is concerned, I know that I can help raise awareness of MG and help obtain funds to support quality research projects that come along. Having myasthenia gravis has impacted my life in many ways. I am totally focused on helping my fellow myasthenics and finding a cure for myasthenia gravis. If through research I could become a small part of making it possible to have a new treatment, even a cure, why I think I'd be so overwhelmed I don't know how I would react!

The Story of Stephen TePastte, M.D.

On the following pages you will find the story of the battle against myasthenia gravis (MG) that is being waged by Dr. Stephen TePastte. Steve is a family physician who practices in Holt, Michigan. This is a town that's a suburb of Lansing—Michigan's capital city and the home of Michigan State University, Steve's alma mater.

Dr. Steve TePastte was stricken with MG in 1998, 19 years after he and a partner founded Holt Family Medicine. Over the years, this practice has added two more family physicians and two physician's assistants. Steve is a popular doctor in Holt. For several consecutive years, he was selected as the town's favorite doctor in surveys of local residents conducted by a local newspaper. He's a physician who is a "people person"—a doctor with a deep understanding of both medicine and people. That understanding is a product of Steve's basic nature furthered by his formal training. Steve earned a master's degree in social psychology at Northwestern University before earning his medical degree at Michigan State. He understands both the "what's" and the "why's" behind what's bothering his patients.

Prior to developing MG, Steve maintained an incredibly fast pace. His days were filled with an overflowing patient-care schedule, family life, and a disciplined dedication to running and working out. The fitness discipline had left him trim and fit and fueled with energy.

The battle Steve TePastte wages against MG has thrust him into an unfamiliar role. In addition to being a doctor, Steve is a patient confronting an often-debilitating chronic disease for which there is management but no cure. This battle has impacted Steve; his wife, Paula, and their daughters, Kelly and Erin; his practice of medicine; and his beliefs and goals. He has embarked on a mission to maintain control of his life and to get the most out of life even in the face of MG. He also has embarked on a mission to guide other chronic disease patients in how to do the same.

Despite the downsides of MG, the story of Steve TePastte is an uplifting one. I have been inspired by his story. Many others, including fellow MG patients, have benefited from what Steve has learned and has taught them about confronting and dealing with a crisis. On the following pages, as Steve recalls his own difficult journey, I think you, too, will find inspiration.

RONALD E. HENDERSON, M.D.

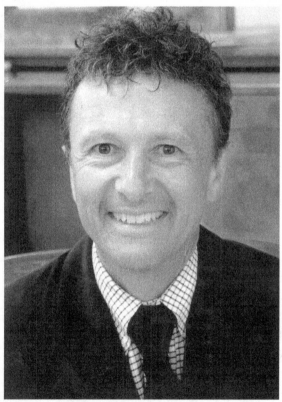

Stephen TePastte, M.D.

13

MUCH MORE THAN DOUBLE VISION

By Stephen TePastte, M.D.

I stood one evening in September 2000 delivering a speech to an audience in Southfield, Michigan, a suburb of Detroit. To deliver the speech, I had driven about 80 miles from where I live and practice family medicine in Holt, Michigan, a suburb of the state's capital city of Lansing.

The Myasthenia Gravis Association there in the Detroit area sponsored the meeting at which I was speaking. This is an organization affiliated with the national Myasthenia Gravis Foundation of America, Inc.

My audience at this meeting—the Association's annual meeting—was made up of 75 to 100 individuals who for one reason or another had a special interest in this rare and little-understood muscle-weakness disease known as myasthenia gravis, or MG. The audience consisted of patients who had been diagnosed with MG, their relatives and friends, and board members of the Myasthenia Gravis Association from various walks of life.

I have been a practicing family physician for two decades and have studied and treated a wide range of diseases. Also, I enjoy making health-related speeches and have spoken on many subjects over the years. However, until recent years myasthenia gravis was not a subject I would have chosen for one of my speeches and was not a subject on which I considered myself an expert.

My interest level in MG was suddenly and unexpectedly heightened in 1998. That's the year I was diagnosed with myasthenia gravis. It was the year I began an insatiable quest for knowledge about this disease, from the point of view of both a patient and a physician.

On that evening in 2000, as I stood and addressed the audience at the Myasthenia Gravis Association near Detroit, my goal was to share some of what I have learned, and to let MG patients and their families in the audience know they were not alone. I was candid about my own experiences with MG. I stood and talked about my own body and how the disease had affected it, about my life and how the disease had affected it, and how I was coping.

I was not prepared for the response I received from the audience. It was overwhelming.

After I finished speaking and had taken some questions from the audience, there was this long line of people from the audience who wanted to talk to me personally. As I talked to them one by one, others waited patiently for their turn. Some of them waited more than an hour.

What I found in talking with these people is that many of them felt confused or even helpless in terms of understanding their MG, in coping with the disease, or both. I talked to individuals who felt there was no one in charge of their disease, no doctor really in charge. I talked to some who just could not understand why things weren't going well for them. Among those with whom I spoke were parents whose children had MG. It was heartbreaking to me, for instance, to see that some of the MG patients there that evening were young girls whose parents were crying about what had happened to their children.

On that evening, I was able to answer some questions, and I was able to share some encouragement. However, that experience made me determined to get even more information on MG—not just for my own family and myself, but also for other MG patients and their families. I remember telling myself, "I have to get *a lot* more information, because this is really powerful stuff. I'm going to make more presentations to help more people. And each time I'm going to know more." I have kept that promise to myself. I have made more presentations on MG, and I will continue to do that.

It occurred to me that I must reach out and help others with MG. I *must*, because for some reason I feel that I have been given an awesome privilege and responsibility to have a strange three-part role, a "triad" if you will, where MG is concerned. First of all, I'm a patient who understands the disease because I have the disease. Secondly, I'm a physician who has a background that enables me to understand and ask questions, to delve into issues at a more-in-depth level than the average lay patient would be likely to do. And thirdly, I really enjoy public speaking and teaching and have been doing that for years. There aren't many MG patients who are surrounded by that triad of circumstances. So to me, I *must* do something for others. I mean, if you're in this situation you're *supposed* to do something.

If that means sharing my own personal story and researching to find answers and options, then that's what I will do. So I speak to the myasthenia patients and their families. I speak about management of myasthenia, about understanding myasthenia, about managing chronic disease and just about fitness and nutrition in general for everyone. All this has created a bond for me—a connection to others who have some circumstances and needs similar to my own.

I'm glad if my own battle against myasthenia gravis helps others.

The "First Inkling"

In my opinion, the prelude to my battle against myasthenia gravis started in the late summer of 1998. To me it started then because that's when the stage was set. I took a little weekend trip with my wife and our younger daughter. It turned out to be a kind of stressful weekend. And not long after that something rare in my life happened: I got sick.

By nature I've always been a driven man and a very healthy, energetic one. My work schedule has been fast-paced, really crazy, ever since my original partner and I founded Holt Family Medicine in 1979. Our practice has been very successful. We've added two other partners and two physician's assistants. We've been very fortunate, because patients have continually gravitated to our office.

Like many doctors, I've probably put in far too many early mornings and late nights and weekends of work. Oh, I managed to squeeze in some time for fitness and running, to which I'm very attached. And I tried to carve out family time, although never nearly enough. Time has been very precious, never quite enough of it.

In late August 1998 I was all set to enjoy this weekend family trip I had afforded myself. At the time, the younger of our two daughters, Erin, was about to begin her senior year in high school and she had a yen for North Carolina. She wanted to go to college there. So my wife, Paula, and I took Erin to North Carolina. There's just a cradle of universities there—Duke, the University of North Carolina at Chapel Hill, etc. We thought, "This is a good chance. We'll fly from Michigan to visit the beautiful state of North Carolina, rent a car and look around and check out colleges for Erin."

The trip had its problems. First of all, Erin got sick. She came down with this really serious gastrointestinal illness, was indisposed, feverish, and felt really bad. Paula and I provided lots of support in order for Erin to see anything. We practically lugged her everywhere we went.

Then there was my "running" mix-up. Wherever I am, I run. I am like this "compulsaholic" fitness guy, into running so much that as of the time we made that trip in 1998 I probably had run 800 days in a row, at least 6 to 8 miles a day. So there we were in North Carolina, and I ventured out to do my daily running. The only problem was that I overran and I got lost. I think I ran three or four hours for like 25 miles total. I really exhausted myself before I found my way.

So, on the heels of Erin getting sick and my getting exhausted with the running, even though I was generally healthy it didn't come as a great surprise to me that a little more than a week later I came down with the same thing Erin had had. I got the virus, too—the fever and gastrointestinal symptoms. It was what I would call a "significant" viral infection.

I got over the virus. But it managed to place my body in a weaker-than-usual state for a time. And I still view that as kind of a preamble, an introduction to what happened next.

What hit me next, actually weeks after the virus, was a vision problem.

I noticed the vision problem one day when I was about to make rounds at the hospital. I thought, "Hey, I'm not seeing really well. I must have my contacts in backwards." But I brushed it off and just forged ahead. I tend to be a "minimalist" and not overreact to stuff. Still, as I was making rounds in the hospital that day, I really had to kind of feel my way around.

After I finished making rounds, I went to a meeting for one of the medical directorships I have (in addition to my medical practice). This meeting was in conjunction with my serving as medical director for a schoolteachers' health insurance program. This is a pretty cool opportunity for me, because I get to do all kinds of wellness programs and websites and public speaking. At any rate, I was attending a meeting for this role; and the vision problem I had just experienced while making hospital rounds worsened. I started seeing two of everybody, and people started drifting further apart in my vision. I was experiencing double vision, technical term *diplopia*. As I sat in the meeting, if I would close one eye when I was looking at an individual I would see only one person; but when I opened both eyes I saw double. Now, this is almost like being blind, unless you close one eye. You don't have any idea which one of the images you're seeing is the real one.

After the meeting, I still continued to forge ahead. I got in my car and started driving to my athletic club. I did this with one eye closed. Since I couldn't see well enough to drive the car, I decided I would park the car and get my bicycle out of the car trunk and ride the bicycle to my destination. The reality of how severe this was had not sunk in with me yet. I got out of the car, and I went to my trunk to get my bike. I realized then that I couldn't function. I was seeing two of *everything*. I couldn't drive the car, and I couldn't ride the bike. I was in trouble. So I called my wife and said, "Paula, I need your help." She thought I had another flat tire. I said, "No, it's not that. Paula, I need your help. I can't drive. I'm seeing double." That was the first inkling.

More Symptoms Lead to Crisis

I was concerned, and Paula was concerned. I mean, one day I seemed fine and the next day I'm having such severe double vision I can't drive a car. What was wrong? My "numbers" were great—cholesterol, blood pressure, etc. I was a fit 50-year-old man who had been healthy all my life. Could I have a brain tumor? Had I suffered a stroke?

Immediately after I experienced the disturbing double vision—later the same day—I saw an ophthalmologist. He told me he thought I just had an eye muscle that was getting a little tired. I sought a second opinion, the same day, from another ophthalmologist. He thought something more serious was going on. He said, "Steve, I think there's something neurologically that's beginning not to work."

So I contacted a neurologist. He ordered a MRI, which I underwent right away. The next day after the double vision hit me I was in the neurologist's office. The MRI came back normal. Although I thought that was fantastic, I knew *something* was wrong.

In the hours that followed, more strange symptoms began to attack my previously healthy body. I was chewing gum, and my chewing muscles stopped working; I couldn't chew it anymore. I was trying to eat, and the food wouldn't go down my throat and I had to spit it out. My speech slowed down, and at times it was garbled. I walked slower, and I began to realize that each time I tried to lift a leg it seemed to take more and more effort. I was so weak I could hardly get out of a chair. I looked terrible. I was wearing this eye patch that the ophthalmologist had prescribed for the double vision. My facial muscles weren't working right and my face was contorted. I went to work, and I saw people there looking at me like they couldn't believe what they were seeing. It was like they were afraid to tell me, "Hey, you look like something is *really, really* wrong with you."

Then came my "day of discovery"—the day when I could go no further without major intervention. It was Friday, December 11, 1998. It had been only two days since it all started. It was on Wednesday of that week when I first experienced the double vision, and here I was on Friday with my condition so deteriorated that I picked up the phone and did the unthinkable for me—I called in to work sick. By that evening, I was sitting at home so incredibly weak I could hardly speak. I was seeing double 100 percent of the time. And I remember that part of a muffin was lodged in my mouth because I couldn't swallow it. My daughter was about to leave the house to go to a rock concert with her friends. I didn't want to burden her with all this stuff, didn't want her to know. So I was anxious that she leave immediately. I believed that very soon I would have to make a trip to a hospital emergency room.

With all this going on, my wife, Paula, looked at me and said, "Steve, your eyes are drooping." Now, Paula is very knowledgeable and observant. She's a nurse who practiced as a nurse for years before entering a second career in retail. Paula noticed the problem with my drooping eyes with very little information from me about what all I had been experiencing. I had not been honest with her, and I had not told her all the symptoms I had been having. When she said, "Your eyes are drooping," it was like a light bulb went on in my brain. It all began to come together, to become clear to me. The drooping eyes, or drooping eyelids, often are a classic early symptom of a rare muscle-weakness disease called myasthenia gravis, or MG. It's one of those so-called "autoimmune diseases" in which the body's immune system seems to turn against an individual. All my symptoms came together and began to make sense. I said, "I have myasthenia gravis."

I telephoned my partners at Holt Family Medicine. They arranged for two neurologists to meet me in the emergency room that evening. They gave me the Tensilon® test—set up an IV and injected the chemical known as Tensilon® into my vein. The deal is that if your symptoms get better when you get Tensilon® that's a pretty good indication that you have myasthenia gravis.

At the beginning, when they gave me the Tensilon® test, I was kind of in my element, as a family doctor who wants to learn, wants to teach. Health professionals that I cared about surrounded me. It was kind of a big deal to watch someone get the Tensilon® test, since myasthenia gravis is a rare disease and you just don't see that many people getting Tensilon®. So I temporarily became the instructor, the teacher. I said, "Now, I want everyone to watch this. This is a teaching case." So they all watched me get better—watched my facial expression come back, watched me lift myself out of my chair and take off my eye patch, and watched me get up and move around. It was confirmed by the Tensilon® test that I had myasthenia gravis.

The only thing Tensilon® is good for at this point is a test to confirm myasthenia gravis. It's not going to stop your symptoms. You get better only temporarily. After I took the Tensilon® test, I actually enjoyed about 20 minutes of major relief before the symptoms began to start again.

In my case, during the next 36 hours, I would get worse, quickly and dangerously.

After my diagnosis was confirmed, the doctors wanted me to spend the night in the hospital. I didn't want to do that. I thought if they would just give me Mestinon®, the medication most used to manage myasthenia gravis symptoms, I could go home and deal with it.

I was released from the emergency room the night of December 11 with prescriptions for Mestinon® and neostigmine. Both are medications to increase muscle strength by blocking an enzyme that's the culprit in causing problems that make the MG patient's muscles weak and non-functional.

However, the medications did not do the job. As the hours wore on, my Mestinon® wasn't working and the neostigmine wasn't helping enough either. I couldn't swallow anything. My ability to swallow was gone entirely. I called one of the neurologists and said, "Look, let's try the injectable stuff." I knew neostigmine can be given by injection and that would get a more concentrated dose into my body. Since Paula is a nurse, she could give me the injections. The doctor was reluctant. He felt I needed to be in the hospital. Reluctantly he agreed to my plan—I was very persistent. He phoned in the injectable neostigmine, and Paula gave me an injection and I went to bed. Paula set an alarm, and every three hours we awakened and she gave me another neostigmine injection.

I knew that instead of getting better I was getting worse. But I was still trying to stay out of the hospital, to manage this thing at home. I thought, "One more injection." Paula gave me the injection. But the swallowing was still a problem. I took a sip of water, and the water just dribbled down my face; it would not go down my throat. My muscles were so weak I could hardly move at all. And the swallowing was such a problem I couldn't even swallow the Mestinon® pills. On Saturday night,

December 12, Paula and I had big social plans. We had been looking forward to attending the annual Christmas party of Holt Family Medicine. Needless to say, we didn't go. In fact, Saturday night was rough. That night I got down nothing—no pills, no food, and no fluids.

By Sunday morning, several things were occurring. One was that I had not urinated at all in about 36 hours; I was getting dehydrated. And I still couldn't swallow at all. But most ominously, I was having trouble moving my chest muscles to breathe. That was the end of the line. I telephoned the neurologist and told him, "I'm ready to go into the hospital. These symptoms are intolerable. I can't function."

As soon as they got me into the hospital, they put in a catheter and tubes, started pumping fluids into me, and gave me not only intravenous neostigmine but also steroids. They also gave me a plasma-exchange treatment called "plasmapheresis" to reduce the amount of problem-causing antibodies in my blood.

For hours I fought the brutal up-and-down battle often experienced by a myasthenic patient in crisis. Everywhere in my body I was feeling this muscle twitching that we call "fasciculation." I endured the side effects of the IV neostigmine, which included tremendous cramps. For an hour the treatment worked great. Then for the next hour and a half it didn't work. My breathing became a major problem. They were talking about putting me on a ventilator. The doctor went out and told my wife, "There is a 99 percent chance that your husband will be intubated overnight. In fact, there's little chance he's going to escape going on the ventilator."

I did escape going on the ventilator, but barely. The neostigmine began to work enough that I could kind of hold my neck up a little and take a few breaths. I think the wellness-focused lifestyle I had practiced over the years helped keep me off that ventilator. I had never been a smoker, I was a dedicated runner and worked out and thus was incredibly fit, and I was very lean. I weighed the same as I weigh now, 130 pounds.

Getting Better and Taking Charge

Gradually after the crisis that December night, I began to get better. The steroids were starting to work. The various other treatments were starting to work. I had 15 to 20 plasmaphereses, and after about four or five of them I was starting to feel pretty good. I was moved out of intensive care onto a regular floor.

I was in the hospital a total of seven days. After I got through the initial crisis, I began sitting up in bed and soaking up information. I was learning and learning and learning about myasthenia gravis. *The more I learned, the more I decided there was little chance I was going to die with this disease; and my goal came to be that I needed to learn to live with the disease.*

I came to realize something. I decided that accepting my diagnosis and focusing on the management of my disease was something I either was going to buy into or not. I mean, this was my life! Was I going to take charge or not? I told myself, "Yes, there's a new captain of managing this disease for me, and I am that captain."

If you're going to be the captain of managing your chronic disease, you need two things: First, you need to feel empowered. That means you need to feel the self-confidence that you have the strength, the power within yourself to have the self-discipline to take care of yourself, and to seek answers and make judgments and decisions about your care. The second thing you need is knowledge. You need to know about your disease.

Since I'm a doctor, it's true that I know more than average about health problems. But a family doctor spends little time studying myasthenia gravis and might never see a case of MG in his or her practice. In fact, at the time I was diagnosed I had never seen a case of myasthenia gravis in the almost 20 years of my practice. At the time I was in the hospital, I knew there were people around me who knew much more about myasthenia gravis than I did. I made it a point to learn from them. I encouraged them to give me knowledge that I was going to need to be the captain, to make decisions about my care, to take care of myself, etc. My point here is you don't have to be a doctor or a nurse or some other type of health professional to become the captain of the management team for your own chronic disease.

While I was there in the hospital, dealing with the aftermath of the diagnosis and that initial crisis, I started gaining the knowledge I needed to run things. Running things does not mean you don't listen to other people. It means you *also* listen to yourself. It means that you approach your disease as a leader and participant, not a follower. Although I look to others to help me, although I have received and continue to receive tremendous help from my physicians, I'm still running things.

Living with the Ups and Downs

It's one thing to be told you have a chronic, incurable disease such as myasthenia gravis. It's another thing to learn to go on with your life despite the limitations that disease brings. The path is seldom easy, but you can find a path. Chronic diseases affect people differently. Some people have severe cases, some much milder ones. With MG, for example, some people might just have the localized form of MG called "ocular MG," limited to weakness of muscles that control eye movements and eyelids. Other MG patients like myself have the more widespread form that affects various muscle groups scattered in the body.

I can tell you from my own experience about the ups and downs of dealing with a chronic disease such as MG: Some days are good. Some days are great. Other days are not so good. The relapses can be challenging. And sometimes the relapses lead to periods of crisis. The key to going forward is to learn to know yourself and your disease, manage yourself wisely, and ride with those ups and downs in a way that you come out on top.

In my case, the first year after I was diagnosed was filled with those ups and downs.

There were more symptoms, plus side effects of some of the medication. It took six months for my eyelids not to droop by the end of the day. Also, I gained weight due to taking prednisone, a steroid medication. Gaining weight was something foreign to me. The weight gain didn't come at the beginning. I remember saying, "You know what? I'm on high dosages of prednisone every day. I don't understand people complaining that steroids make you gain weight. It hasn't done that to me." Well, I spoke too soon. Two weeks after I said that I had gained 20 pounds. Then the weight gain totaled 30 pounds, and then 40. I was puffy in the face, and I weighed more than I had ever weighed in my life, much more.

I also had to have more treatment. Five months after my initial diagnosis and crisis, I underwent surgery to remove my thymus gland. This is a surgical procedure called a thymectomy. The thymus gland, which lies behind the breastbone, is part of our immune system and is thought to be defective when you develop myasthenia gravis. Some but not all of MG patients undergo the thymectomy. Some but not all of those who undergo a thymectomy will experience some improvement in their MG condition.

That year of 1999, the year after my diagnosis, also held several months of feeling pretty good. Life returned to full and productive. I was able to get back to work—not on the same rigorous schedule I had kept before, but nevertheless back and active. I was back to running and working out. I was able to taper down on the steroid treatment, and my weight was getting back in line.

Then, before 1999 came to an end, I suffered a major relapse. In the early fall of 1999 I got a virus. About six weeks later, beginning on a Saturday in late October, I had a relapse. It came almost 11 months after my initial diagnosis. On that October Saturday afternoon, I was playing golf. It was an odd treat in Lansing, Michigan, to have weather nice enough to play golf that late in the fall. I was playing with a friend. And all of a sudden what I was seeing was a fuzzy ball—sort of fuzzy and kind of a half ball. Then I was seeing two balls, and I didn't know which one to hit. Most of the time that afternoon I was hitting at the wrong ball, the one that wasn't there, and my real ball was just going everywhere. I knew all too well what my problem had to be, but I didn't tell my friend. Playing golf obviously wasn't working. Finally my friend just joked with me and said, "Hey, I'm leaving. There are too many bad golfers on the course." The next day, Halloween, it was worse. I was seeing double so badly that it seemed to me there were far more trick-or-treaters around than there should have been. It was like I woke up and it—the MG—was all back. In 24 to 36 hours I had gone from feeling okay as far as I could tell, to feeling almost as bad as when I had been in the hospital the previous December. With my doctor's help, we got me over that. We increased the steroids again. We did the plasmapheresis.

I was able to get back to work. But it took me six months to really get back to where I had been. I had had trouble swallowing all along since I got myasthenia gravis, and for a while after the relapse the swallowing problems got pretty bad. My face didn't want to work. My eye muscles didn't want to work. And I will admit that during that six months there were periods when I got really frustrated, discouraged, and dispirited. I didn't get depressed as much as I got scared—scared because I love life so much. I was scared that I wasn't going to be able to be back to where I wanted to be, scared of loss of functionality, of not being able to have my life. When you're a myasthenia patient, at times you can feel that your life is lost.

However, I focused on what I had committed to myself that I would do within days of my diagnosis—that is, to take a leading role in managing my disease. I worked with my doctor. I took care of myself. I tried to focus on the positive. Gradually, I got better and more and more active.

As I relate this story in December 2001, I'm proud to report that I have not suffered a major relapse since that one on the golf course in the fall of 1999. That's two good years of carefully managing my disease and taking in life.

Some Good Along with the Bad

If you speak long enough with any chronic disease patient who is successfully coping with his or her disease, I think the patient will tell you that even with all the "bad" the disease has brought, there also has been some "good."

I believe this happens because, if you cope successfully with your disease, you have no choice but to take a long look at the way you were living your life prior to this disease, rethink what you value most, set priorities, and make necessary changes. After all, the two-fold goal of any positive-thinking chronic disease patient is (1) to manage your disease as best it can be managed, and (2) to continue to live as productive a life as possible.

If your experience is anything like mine, as you confront your life in the face of a chronic disease, as you decide about values, priorities and changes, you will experience a renewal.

You will retain some of the good in your life, discard some of the bad, and make some pleasant discoveries along the way.

Below are key areas in which some "good" has come about in my life since I was diagnosed with myasthenia gravis three years ago.

"Restructuring" on the Work Front

I still work as a doctor, but I have modified how that work is structured. In making these modifications, I'm now doing the doctoring things I care about most.

When I first got sick, I had to be off work for two months. For a short time I considered going on disability. Then I decided against it. On the one hand, I realized that MG and the treatments I was taking to control MG had changed my professional picture somewhat, that the changes meant that I could not do all the things I once did. On the other hand, I felt I was not too sick to work within a reasonable structure. So I went about putting that structure together.

You see, I love practicing medicine. I love it so much I'd virtually do it for free. I love our practice, Holt Family Medicine. After all, I was one of the founders of that practice. This is a family practice in which I take incredible pride. It's one of the last of a breed—fully independent, private, and not affiliated with a health-system group. Our practice has a wonderful teaching affiliation with the medical school faculty at my alma mater there in East Lansing, Michigan State University. Holt Family Medicine is a place where patients get top-notch care, where the doctors and other staff have motivation and principles guided by making the patient well and being as straight with the patients as you can get.

So now I'm back at work at Holt Family Medicine, in a different structure that addresses the reality of myasthenia gravis but still enables e to be productive and help patients. Because I am taking steroid medication—immunosuppressant medication that suppresses my immune system and makes me susceptible to contagious diseases—I no longer see "sick" patients at the office. If someone comes in with a cold or a virus, that patient is referred to one of my physician partners or one of our physician's assistants. I no longer make hospital rounds. I don't spend as much time at Holt Family Medicine as I formerly did, and I don't take as many patients as I formerly did. As things stand now, I am so overbooked during the time I am there I cannot take any new patients.

But there is good that has come out of these changes—good for me and good for my patients. I now spend virtually all my patient-care time doing something I feel my patients really need and what I think I do best—working with wellness, lifestyle issues, disease management, and problem solving. I always emphasized those areas even prior to getting MG. Now I focus totally on them. Ever since I started practicing medicine, I've felt that my psychology background (bachelor's degree in psychology, master's degree in social psychology) was one of the reasons I've had so many patients. My basic nature makes me delve into what's really bothering patients. I've always tried to work with my patients in addressing the problems in their lives, in living healthier lives. I really enjoy people and love my patients. Each one of them is my friend. When a patient comes into my office, I welcome that patient with a hug. Man, woman, child, young adult, middle-aged person, grandma, whatever, that patient is my friend. Even in the old days, prior to MG, back when I was involved in the whole spectrum of patient care, I would ask patients about underlying problems. If a patient came in with a sprained ankle and also appeared to be worried about more than the ankle, I would try to identify the reason for the patient's worry. I would say, "Well, yeah, we'll stick an Ace wrap and an ice pack on this ankle, and then you can sit down and tell me what's really going on in your life."

These days at Holt Family Medicine I'm focusing more on those kinds of things, on wellness and lifestyle issues in which I really take pride. I take pride in helping someone quit smoking, in guiding someone in how to patch up a marriage, in helping a patient feel empowered to take ownership of his or her disease, in teaching the high blood pressure patient how to get that blood pressure under control, and teaching the diabetic how to manage his or her disease. Those kinds of things get me excited.

As I have cut back on the amount of time I spend at Holt Family Medicine, I've begun devoting a significant amount of my work time to, and earning a good percentage of my income from, some "medical directorships" I have. I'm medical director of an insurance company, medical director of a health program for teachers, and medical director of a community education program. Also I consult on wellness and life insurance programs for a corporation. All these things bring diversity to my work. I'm teaching wellness, disease management. In conjunction with these roles, I'm working with websites, writing health brochures, and speaking on health topics.

I also make sure I structure my life so there's time left for my new volunteer role. This role is through the Myasthenia Gravis Association. I speak to and answer questions of MG patients and their families and also physicians, residents, and medical students who want to learn more about MG.

For me the message out of all of this is yes, my chronic disease has brought change to my professional life. But these changes aren't all bad—far from it. There's a lot of good here.

Closer Family Ties

There is no doubt in my heart and mind that since I was diagnosed with MG I've become closer to my wife and two daughters, Erin, 21, and Kelly, 25.

Paula, my wife, is incredible, in so many ways.

My relationship with Paula goes back a little more than 30 years. I met her not long after I decided to become a doctor but before I entered medical school. I had just received my master's degree in social psychology from Northwestern; and I was back in Lansing taking courses at my undergraduate alma mater, Mchigan State University. My goal was to be accepted into medical school there. While I was taking these courses, I was earning some money and exposing myself to a medical environment by working as a hospital orderly. This was a job that mostly meant I either was putting in catheters or carrying bodies down to the hospital morgue. One day while working at the hospital, I found myself in the operating room with a young student nurse named Paula. The surgery in progress was one in which the surgeon "pins back" the ears of someone whose ears stick out too far—a procedure called otoplasty. Something about this procedure didn't sit well with Paula. She fainted. I rushed to her rescue. We got to know one another. One thing led to another, and ultimately we married. I tease a bit as I look back; I say that I rushed to the rescue of Florence Nightingale and then I married her.

One thing that still is significant to me about our courtship is that Paula accepted and fell in love with a hospital orderly, not a doctor. Oh, it's true my goal was to enter medical school, but goals don't always convert to reality. Paula accepted me as I was then, and she believed in me.

When I say that Paula is incredible, I say that partly because Paula is a person who has powerful strength. You might not see that strength when you first meet her. She's so sweet. That's what you might notice first. But that strength is there, too. She's also very disciplined. Paula and I share a love of fitness, of running, of working out. Paula is trim and fit, as fit a woman as you'll ever meet at any age. And she's tough. During one period when she was running very hard every day for about 5 to 6 miles, she broke both legs while running—suffered stress fractures in both legs—and for a time she didn't even realize her legs were fractured.

Despite the wonderful woman, wife, and mother Paula has been through the years, I think prior to my having MG we didn't communicate as well as we should have. I think we didn't spend enough time together. I was working so hard and was so driven. After a rigorous, non-stop day, when I finally did make it home, it was more convenient for me just to sit downstairs and watch a football or basketball game on TV, to crash. I wasn't paying enough attention to my wife; I was not spending enough time with her.

We have these two bright, beautiful daughters of whom we're both so proud. Erin is a junior at the University of North Carolina in Chapel Hill. Kelly is a teacher in Honduras, teaching English to Hondurans, with plans to return to The States for graduate school. While I always have been close to the girls, I credit Paula with so much of the "nitty-gritty" of their rearing. And she did a wonderful job. I think for many years I carried out an unfair role with those two girls. When I was with them, I talked to them about blue sky, education, purpose in life, fitness and having fun. But someone in the household had to deal with the day-to-day issues. Paula was good at that, and it was easy for me to let Paula do that. Whenever there was tension, I left that to Paula. It was like, "Hey, it wasn't me (who said this or that, or took a given position on something)."

My battle against myasthenia gravis has strengthened my relationship with Paula; it has strengthened our marriage. Paula has lent me unwavering support through all this. Her unwavering support dates back to Day One. That was the day when I was having double vision, had no idea what was wrong, and telephoned her to say, "Paula, I need your help. I can't drive."

I've come to really appreciate, probably to an extent I never would have without MG, how very important it is to have a life mate. I love and appreciate Paula, and, like I said, she's incredible.

Putting Stress in Perspective

I don't know to what degree stress plays a role in myasthenia gravis—or any other chronic disease. But I think it does play a role. Stress that's out of control, that's making a person chronically tense and anxious, likely helps trigger some illnesses and diseases. Also, stress that's out of control likely makes some illnesses and diseases worse after you get them. *I think it's safe to say, both from my view as a doctor and as a chronic disease patient, that management of stress is a key element in managing my disease.*

Now, we all have some stress in our lives. You can't live your life and confront issues and problems and deal with them without having some stress. However, you can reduce your stress level. You can give thought to stress in your life and how you can best deal with it. You can to some extent reduce your stress and at least make choices about what you worry about and what you don't worry about, and how you drive yourself and where to pull back.

I think I had far too much stress in my life prior to being diagnosed with myasthenia gravis. As to whether that stress played a role in my getting MG I can't say. *I can say that it has been necessary for me to reduce and manage that stress in order to manage the MG.*

Some of the stress I faced prior to MG was a natural by-product of the busy, pressured life I lived. Some of the stress I brought on myself. I was very driven. I think I was too concerned about working very hard and saving for retirement. I drove myself too much and I worried too much about the future. I mean, looking back I think it was a dumb thing for me to focus on the stock market ticker so much. I would go to the athletic club and just sit and watch that thing! Now, why would I want to worry and focus on that all the time? If you have investments, you should look at your portfolio every now and then; but day-to-day monitoring will drive you crazy. That's true of a lot of other things in life, too.

All in all, I think I was unnecessarily driving myself a little crazy then. To be blunt, I think I had filled my life with a lot of worry that I needed to get rid of.

Having myasthenia gravis has made me reflect a lot on what my life is about. While I'm doing my solitary running, whatever has happened during that day gets filtered against this list of what I call my own special "true order" of what's most important. And usually what happens is that so many things turn out not to be important at all. I just say, "Well, why did I bother about that? Who cares about that?" And I forget about it.

Reflecting on my Roots

I think there are some people in life that you value and appreciate before you get sick, and then *after* you get sick you value and appreciate them even more.

That's the case with how I feel about my parents. Since I was diagnosed with myasthenia gravis, I've had to call on all the strength I could find within myself, and then strive to make myself even stronger. My parents planted seeds of strength in my two younger brothers and me, and I thank them for that.

My brothers and I are fortunate that we still have our parents, both in their 80s, doing really well physically, and, as always, doing incredibly well emotionally, spiritually, and intellectually. They still make their home in the Michigan city where I grew up, Grand Rapids.

I thank my parents for what they are and for always being there for my brothers and me.

Our creative father—craftsman, interior decorator, artist who has created lovely oil paintings, and now also photography expert—was always a very hands-on dad. In fact, he was my Little League coach. I always told people that if you were going to lie to my dad, Gerrit TePastte, you'd better have a very good memory. My dad will track your story, and if you lie to him you're going to have to keep changing your story to make it work. And it *still* won't work. My dad is rock-solid, high-intellect, incredibly honest, and straightforward.

As for our mother, Mary TePastte, she was very loved at the college where she worked for years. On one occasion when she was ill and they were holding a special reunion at the college, they just turned the event into an appreciation for her! At the college, where she was a dean's secretary, she touched people with the same trait that was felt so much by my brothers and me as we grew up. Everyone who has ever met my mother has been touched by the fact that she made them feel they were something special, someone who had a special purpose in life, and someone who was supposed to do something. The thing my mother gave to all three of her sons was a sense of making us feel special. That was my mother's gift to my brothers and me.

Spirituality

Spirituality means so many things to so many different people. Different spiritual views. Different faiths and denominations. Different ways of "practicing" and "exercising" one's spirituality.

I have grown in spirituality since MG came into my life.

When I was growing up, my brothers and I attended the Baptist church some. But even though I went there as a kid, and even though I saw some things in the church that impressed me positively, I don't think I ever really took acceptance of all the teachings. One of the things that did impress me positively was seeing that the church was a powerful, wonderful organization that did a tremendous amount of good for many people in need. I saw how much the church helped people, how the people in the church would rally around those in need, such as those who were sick. I saw how church members' spirit, faith, and prayer seemed to make them stronger.

But as I grew into adulthood and went on living my life, much of what I had been exposed to in the church really was not a driving force for me. It was not something that I thought that much about—until I got myasthenia gravis.

Keep in mind that I really never had been sick, or really in crisis, until all those MG symptoms descended on me so rapidly. Then, there I was very sick at age 50, in the hospital emergency room and then in intensive care. Having never been in a similar situation, as my condition worsened and I couldn't breathe and all this activity was going on around me, it took awhile for it to register with me how serious this was. It took awhile for me to confront the fact that this really was *me* in this situation and that the situation was dismal. But reality did dawn. I saw that my wife was crying. And my mom was crying. The doctor, who was like 6 feet, 8 inches tall and just this big bear of a man, was a friend of mine. And *he* came in and was crying. I was kind of getting nervous. I'm thinking, "Well, maybe I won't live." You know, if you're in that situation it stands to reason that a sort of twang of spirituality might come then. And for me it sort of came then.

Then there was the prayer issue. While I was lying there in intensive care, all these people began praying for me. Some who prayed were my friends and patients, people I knew. Others were people I had never met. Word had spread quickly about my being sick. For example, after I was admitted to the hospital on Sunday, patients of Holt Family Medicine were asking a lot of questions the next day. My not being at work was an unusual event. I mean, I had missed very little work in 20 years. The office switchboard lit up. My patients were asking, "Where is Dr. TePastte? You cancelled my appointment with him on Friday because he was not at work, and now he's not here again today. What's really going on?" As I've already said, in our practice we shoot straight with our patients. So my patients were told the truth: "He's in intensive care. He's almost on a ventilator." My patients have always been kind of like my family. They started sending these get-well cards to me at the hospital. Those cards just poured in. Why, I probably received a total of 2,000 to 3,000 cards, many of them from my patients. And in those cards so many people talked about prayer and told me that their church was praying for me. Now, I didn't go to any of their churches. But all these churches in the whole South Lansing community were praying for me. And they kept praying for me. They kept praying and praying and praying. And, after being so sick, gradually I got to feeling pretty good. I began wondering about this prayer issue. I'm thinking, "Let's look into this."

So I actually did my own research about prayer. I learned that Duke University had conducted a study in which they divided some heart patients into two groups. In one group, the caregivers prayed for the patients. In the other group, the caregivers did not pray for the patients. And the heart patients didn't know about who was being prayed for and who wasn't. As it turned out, the patients who were prayed for did a lot better.

Well, this impressed me. I was thinking, "I owe a tremendous amount of gratitude to all those people who prayed for me, because I really do think they helped to make me better." Now, I don't think that the prayer was the only thing. I received some good care. Also, I think what's inside you, the individual, is significant. I think what's right inside your heart is important.

But I do think that a Super Being created me, that He has given me tremendous powers, and that I myself must use those powers to stay in control of my destiny. He has given me tremendous freedoms. I feel super-empowered and super-in-control in the sense of my destiny.

All in all, since I've had MG I think I have become more of a spiritual person. And I think I've become much more effective as a physician. Today I teach people about spirituality and feeling empowered. I listen to their own beliefs, their own view of spirituality; and I try to work with them in utilizing their spirituality for empowerment that helps them deal better with their health and their overall lives.

Messages for Patients

When you have a chronic disease such as myasthenia gravis, you have to find that magic recipe of medications and other treatments that works best for you. The same is true in finding a healthy regimen of lifestyle practices that meets your needs. Approaching the management of a chronic disease is not a case of "one size fits all." There must be an individual approach to each individual patient's situation.

I know some things that have worked for me. They make up a list I share with other myasthenia gravis patients when I speak to them. I want to share my list with you as food for thought as you and your doctors work together in finding your own path to managing your disease.

Although I'm listing these with myasthenia gravis in mind, I think in several areas there are general thoughts that apply to patients with various other chronic diseases as well.

1. **Take control of your disease.** Realize that myasthenia gravis is a "snowflake" disease—that each case of MG, like each snowflake, is different. Be knowledgeable about MG and your options in treatment. Be proactive, not passive, in seeking answers, in making judgments about your care. Keep in mind that no one treatment fits all.

2. **Approach your disease as though you are in a partnership with your doctor—keeping in mind that *you* are the partner in charge.** I think it's okay to refer to this doctor-and-patient relationship as a "partnership." But somebody has to be in charge. And the doctor should not be the one in charge. The patient should be in charge. The doctor works for the patient. One of the doctor's roles is to empower the patient with knowledge and hopefully to help the patient understand the power of assertiveness and taking ownership. As a patient, look at it this way: Ask yourself if you would give your money to a retirement planner and say, "Hey, you're the retirement planner, don't tell me anything, you go ahead and do it. I don't want to know." Then ask yourself the extent to which you are involved in managing your own healthcare. Why in the world would you not want to be deeply involved with something that important? If you're leaving everything up to the doctor and not learning about your health problems and not participating, you should be telling yourself, "What the hell am I doing, passively dealing with my own health? Am I crazy

or what?" I have a little tip for you in dealing with your doctor: When an uncertain situation comes up about your health, such as which way to go with your treatment, ask your doctor, "What would *you* do in this situation?"

3. Recognize the power you have within yourself. I've already discussed how important I feel this is. Be self-confident about managing your chronic disease. Believe in your rights and your knowledge as a patient. Those things empower you. If you don't have enough knowledge, get some more.

4. Take your medicines. If you think you can stop your medicines, or that you can just take them every now and then, you're going to get into trouble. There's never an excuse to not take your medicine. I never miss my medicine.

5. Before taking herbs and vitamin supplements, check them out with your doctor. Make sure your doctor knows you are taking them. I make speeches on the subject of herbs and supplements. This is one of my interests. While I believe some herbs and supplements can be helpful to certain individuals in certain situations, I also can tell you that some of these things are very potent, very powerful. Some can make you bleed, raise your blood pressure, create heart rhythm disturbances, and stimulate your immune system in a way it might not need to be stimulated—just to name a few possibilities. In discussing herbs and vitamin supplements with your doctor, make sure a given herb or supplement that has attracted your interest will not adversely interact with your prescription medicines or create conditions in your body that could put you at risk. In my personal situation with myasthenia gravis, the only vitamins I take are those that I recommend for my patients.

6. Exercise if you can. Unless there is a medical reason that prevents your exercising, I would recommend that you do it. Before you proceed, talk to your doctor about you and exercise. I have exercised for years and I think it has helped me overall in my life. I strongly feel exercise continues to help me in managing myasthenia gravis. There's no doubt in my mind that I was able to better sustain blows dealt me by myasthenia gravis because my body had been so conditioned and strengthened over the years by regular, rigorous exercise. In fact, I love exercise so much that I have to watch myself so that I don't overdo it. So what is it about exercise that's so great? Many things. Part of it is spiritual, because you feel powerful. Part of it is psychological, because you feel in control. You get this positive feedback that your body is okay. Part of it is relieving stress. Part of it involves the proteins called endorphins that are released; and these endorphins, among other good things, actually are analgesic—that is, pain-relieving. Part of it is your heart is stronger. Part of it is your blood vessels are stronger and you get better circulation to those areas you're exercising. Part of it is you metabolize glucose better and you become insulin-sensitive, not insulin-resistant. It's *everything*. Every single component of your body is better. Specifically where exercise and myasthenia gravis are concerned, I've found that the fitness part of myasthenia gravis is something so many people don't want to talk about. I personally think that's nuts. You read some of the information on MG, and basically the message about exercise comes across something like, "Well, yeah, I guess you can work out, but you better check, maybe go see a rehab doc." It is my opinion that exercise greatly helps many MG patients. Of course, you should do it in a safe manner. But I feel you've got to challenge yourself and do it and move a little bit further every day. If you can, make yourself do it.

7. **Prepare for relapses.** When you have a chronic disease, there is no guarantee that you won't get a relapse. You must prepare yourself emotionally for that. In the case of myasthenia gravis, not only is there no guarantee you won't get a relapse; there's a pretty good chance you *will* get one. And the truth is there is no guarantee if you get a relapse that you're going to overcome it to the degree you would like to. Just take care of yourself, enjoy every day, and prepare to roll with the punches.

8. **If possible, do not quit work and go on disability because you have myasthenia gravis or some other chronic disease. Try to prevent what I refer to as "rewarding yourself for being sick."** I want to make it clear here that I know there are some patients who have health problems so severe that quitting work and going on disability is the only option. However, my advice to patients with chronic health problems is to continue some type of work whenever possible. You might find you have to restructure your work, that you need to do things a bit differently from what you did prior to having this chronic health problem. That might mean taking a less stressful approach to your old line of work, or changing your line of work totally. It might mean part-time work instead of full-time work. The bottom line is that it's so important to be active and to feel productive. I have told some of my patients, "I want you to try to avoid getting rewarded for being sick. Because if you're rewarded for being sick, I can't make you well. I'm not against disability payments and compensation. I understand it, and it's necessary insurance. But if you need to be sick to get paid, I can't make you well."

9. **Participate in and support a chapter of a health organization or support group for those with your chronic health problem.** There you will gain knowledge through speeches and seminars. There you will meet others in a similar situation and share knowledge and mutual support. There you will find avenues to join forces with others in helping needy patients who have the same problem you do. In many of these organizations, you also will find an opportunity to band together with others to support research aimed at learning more about the health problem that affects you. *To myasthenia gravis patients, I say, "Participate in and support a chapter of the Myasthenia Gravis Foundation—the people who care about you and your disease, the people who support you."*

Messages for Doctors

In giving advice to the medical community about myasthenia gravis, my messages are few but specific:

1. No matter what your specialty might be as a doctor, learn about the symptoms of myasthenia gravis. You might never see a case in your entire practice. However, you might see several cases. And you can save a lot of suffering, heartbreak, and emotional distress on the part of a MG patient if you're able to pick up on MG symptoms soon after a patient presents them. Many MG patients are sent to psychiatrists because doctors think the symptoms sound so strange and unrelated that they must be in the patient's head. For example, knowing about MG could help you at least consider MG as a possible answer if a patient comes to you complaining of weak eyelid muscles, slurred speech, chewing or swallowing problems, and weakness in the arms or legs. Or an undiagnosed MG patient might come in complaining of muscle weakness in other parts of the body. Myasthenia gravis has such a variety of muscle-weakness symptoms, and several different patients with MG could come in with several sets of symptoms.

2. Be honest with your patients. This is a real issue with me, whether you're dealing with MG or some other problem. It takes a great amount of skill and also some courage to be totally up-front with patients. But it's your *duty* to do that. Be as honest with the patient as you would if that patient was your wife or husband, your mother or father. If you don't know what's wrong with the patient, tell the patient. Try to find out what's wrong yourself, or refer the patient to someone you think can find out what's wrong. As a physician, recognize the limits of your ability in a specific situation; know when to refer the patient to another physician. I have never felt a negative reaction from a patient by just looking the patient in the eye, being sincere, and saying, "There's something wrong with you. I don't know yet what it is. We've got to figure out what it is." A patient often is relieved to hear that. For then the patient is comforted by the fact that, even if the doctor does not know what's wrong, the doctor believes there really is a problem and is trying to help the patient.

3. Treat the patient as an individual and arrive at a treatment regimen that is tailored to that patient's needs. Don't try to use the same treatment regimen for every person who has the same diagnosis. To individualize and tailor treatment, you must take time to know your patient. You must listen to your patient, and you must talk to your patient. I know all too well how important it is to have an individualized approach for myasthenia gravis patients. That's true with many other chronic diseases as well.

4. Teach the patient how to become a partner in managing his or her chronic health problems, whether the patient has myasthenia gravis or some other health problem. Work with the patient in paving the way for the patient to take ownership of his or her healthcare. Do your part in creating that doctor/patient "partnership."

A Daughter's View

If you're suffering from a serious chronic health problem, it requires a lot of your energy and attention to focus on managing that problem and also continuing to live a productive life. I know.

However, as we go about balancing chronic disease and living life, it's important that we not become too self-absorbed. We must look beyond ourselves and be aware of, be sensitive to, what's going on with our loved ones, particularly our close family members such as our spouses, children, parents, and siblings.

A chronic disease has the power to bring about immense stresses and changes in the lives of the patient. That chronic disease also has the power to bring about immense stresses and changes in the lives of the patient's loved ones.

My younger daughter, Erin, was 17 years old when I was diagnosed. Along with my wife, Paula, our older daughter, Kelly, my parents, and other members of our family, Erin went through tremendous turmoil in watching her usually very active and healthy dad suddenly placed in harm's way by myasthenia gravis.

Erin has the ability to put her feelings on paper. She was 18 when she wrote the following essay for a college English class. This essay gives insight into her feelings and anxieties about my battle against myasthenia gravis. She wrote this in late May 2000, almost 18 months after I was diagnosed. By this time I had been "to hell and back" so to speak, having been critically ill, then better, then through a relapse, and better again. In an essay she entitled "A Rare Disease, a Step into Reality," these are the words of Erin TePastte:

Having a family physician in the family improved my understanding of disease. Disease was something that happened to people who lead an unhealthy or high-risk lifestyle; not a family that exercises every day, rarely drinks, and whose eating habits include the most important food groups. I've never worried about medications or vaccinations because as soon as anyone felt a symptom, my Dad would rush home. But in December of 1998, my Dad couldn't rush home. In fact, he couldn't see to drive home because he was seeing double. The "wellness" leader in my life was headed for an unsuspected challenge.

At first we suspected a tumor, but after he started experiencing other strange symptoms, we were scared and confused about what it was. After his vision went, he also began to lose his speech, and then his arm and leg muscles became extremely weak. The next day he couldn't swallow or open his eyes, so my mother checked him into the hospital where he diagnosed himself with a rare disease called Myasthenia Gravis. His patients, family and friends were astonished to hear the tragic news because he plays such a major role in all of their lives. Basically anyone who comes in contact with this five-foot, six-inch energetic man falls in love. His passion for life, and his ability to help others love themselves by treating their bodies right, made him irresistible. Consequently, the sad news was a test of his true passion for life.

The news of this disease didn't hit me until I saw him in the hospital. The man who was a symbol of life to me lay weak and sad, with tubes entering and exiting every orifice. I couldn't speak. I had nothing to say. I just stared at what seemed to be my father, completely flabbergasted to what my mind was slowly coming to grips with. Could he die?

"It's treatable," some distant voice echoes to reassure me.

"He looks bad, but this disease allows a full recovery," some other almost imaginary voice stirs into my ears.

During the time he was in the hospital, I wanted to be there, but at the same time, I wanted to distance myself from a feared truth: goodbye. Even though family, friends, and even doctors (including my Dad) reassured me he would be fine, I couldn't believe it until he was home, running around the house. I realized how much I don't trust other people's words, even my Dad's. He would mutter that he was going to be all right, but by looking at the tubes and machines and hearing his slurred voice, it didn't comprehend. Through this experience, I found out how weak I really was, and I learned to never underestimate the strength of my mother. I normally view myself as a positive person, but this event proved that in times of uncertainty my glass was definitely half-empty.

Myasthenia Gravis (MG) is an autoimmune disease. Autoimmune disease is caused by an error in our immune system. The immune system normally functions to protect us from diseases caused by infections. To protect ourselves against recurrent diseases, our immune system can form antibodies that kill the invading organism on contact. Hence, we only get common infections like Chicken Pox and Mononucleosis once. In autoimmune illnesses, the immune system mistakenly forms an antibody against our own healthy tissue. In MG sufferers the immune system attacks muscle enzymes leading to severe weakness. Myasthenia Gravis is Latin for "severe muscle weakness."

MG is rare, with an incidence of about one per 25,000 people; but the family of autoimmune disease is quite common. Other more familiar autoimmune disorders include many kinds of arthritis and most thyroid disturbances. No one knows why someone gets an autoimmune disease. They are not contagious or inheritable. It is best to consider the cause to be an accident of nature that occurs randomly.

My father thinks that his immune system may have been over-stimulated by excess exercise. Vigorous exercise is healthy for the immune system, but exhausting exercise can be harmful. Mostly though, he feels the illness just happened randomly for no specific reason. He feels that about 80 percent of disease is preventable by a healthy lifestyle. Heart attacks, strokes, and most cancers are common examples of preventable diseases. The other 20 percent are probably not preventable, but you can prepare yourself to overcome them.

My father believes that the life he leads has prepared him to successfully battle this chronic disease. Despite a prescribed long and strenuous, but full recovery, my Dad achieved a speedy, full recovery in two months. By then, he was back to his hectic schedule of patients, emergency rooms, insurance agencies, and twenty-five mile bike rides. Even before he regained full use of his muscles, the most important muscle was never defeated: his smile.

This sudden obstacle in my Dad's life, I experienced second-hand, but in a bitter reality which made me feel guilty. How terribly lucky I am, so healthy and loved, swimming in the stupidity of my perfect world; when the biggest piece of my perfect world became a statistic, a statistic of the small part of the population that has Myasthenia Gravis. Since my Dad is so incredibly healthy both mentally and physically, he's recovered like he never had the disease in the first place. The perfect world returns, only this time, as I'm enjoying the life of being the lucky daughter of the TePasttes, I look behind me every once-in-awhile to see if reality will catch up again.

The Story of J. Steven Gaines, Ph.D.

The story that follows is one of persistence, tenacity, and acceptance made possible by exceptional spiritual faith. It is the story of Dr. Steve Gaines, high-profile Baptist minister and also myasthenia gravis patient.

Dr. Gaines is the senior pastor of Gardendale's First Baptist Church. This is a church located in the Birmingham, Alabama, suburb of Gardendale—a church that is one of the largest and fastest-growing Baptist churches in the state of Alabama.

On the following pages, as you learn of Dr. Gaines' battle against MG, I believe you will be inspired, as I have been, by his strength and determination. In spite of the challenges MG has brought into his life, Dr. Gaines continues to lead an active life as senior pastor. In his story, Dr. Gaines explains how a reorganization of his church's ministerial team has helped him to continue to lead and still have the strength and stamina to preach four sermons each Sunday. He describes the powerful support he has received from his family, friends, and church family. He reveals how walking the path of a MG patient has led him to form an even closer bond with God.

A forthright man who faces life head-on, Dr. Steve Gaines wasted no time after his diagnosis before he stood in the pulpit and shared his news with members of his congregation. He told them he had this rare disease called MG. He explained that as a related development of the MG he also had a tumor on his thymus gland, that he must undergo surgery to have his thymus gland removed, and that this meant he would be absent for a few weeks from the pulpit.

When Dr. Gaines stands in the pulpit on Sunday morning, he reaches his own large church congregation plus thousands more via an extended television audience. Each Sunday, his sermon is televised on one of Birmingham's leading television stations. Thus, after Steve Gaines was diagnosed with MG, word spread quickly. Many who had never heard of MG were hearing that a highly visible local minister in the prime of life now was battling this rare disease.

By continuing his ministry despite MG, Dr. Gaines is in a unique position to show by example what one can accomplish by accepting a condition, putting it on a back shelf, and focusing on the job ahead. It is my privilege to call Steve Gaines my friend and fellow Christian.

RONALD E. HENDERSON, M.D.

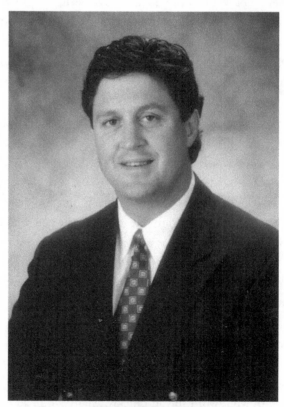

J. Steven Gaines, Ph.D.

14

A New View from the Pulpit

By J. Steven Gaines, Ph.D.

When I left with my family for a vacation trip to California in July 2000, I felt I was in deep need of this period of rest and relaxation—much more so than with just the average vacation.

My wife and children and I had planned ahead for two full weeks of sightseeing and family fun in San Diego, Los Angeles, and San Francisco. I was excited, and so were they. For two weeks, none of us would have any commitments except to enjoy one another. All of my immediate family came along. With me were Donna, my wife of 20 years; and our four children—son, Grant; and daughters, Lindsey, Allison, and Bethany, at the time ages 17, 13, 11, and 6, respectively.

I naturally was looking forward to the two weeks of family togetherness. In our family, we enjoy one another's company and we do a lot of things together. Also, I was looking forward to a relaxing background in which to reflect on and pray about the stressful events in my life during the past several weeks and months.

I had several things to sort out, both personally and professionally.

In my personal life, it was an especially challenging time. It had been only a month since my father had died. I had just learned that my mother had been diagnosed with breast cancer. My only sibling, my brother, Ed, was getting a divorce after years of marriage.

In my professional life, I had issues to work through in my role as the senior pastor of a large and rapidly growing Baptist church located in the community of Gardendale, Alabama, a suburb of Birmingham. Because our church has grown so rapidly, it has outgrown our current facilities. At the time my family and I went to California in the summer of 2000, the church was in the planning stages of a massive expansion. However, we were running into major obstacles procuring the land we needed to go forward with that expansion.

Then there was the mysterious problem of my declining physical strength. Up until around early 1999, all my life I had been very healthy and physically strong. But something had gone wrong. I didn't know what it was. I just felt tired—very, very tired. In fact, I felt that way most of the time. I felt a general overall loss of energy and stamina. For months now I had hoped this was temporary and would get better. But the truth of the matter was that the fatigue had stayed with me for longer than I cared to admit—for about 18 months at this point. Also, instead of getting better, the fatigue was steadily getting worse. In truth, the fatigue had become so severe it was limiting my activities and more and more could be considered debilitating. By the time I went on vacation, I was feeling the fatigue and the current stresses in my life to the point I was just flat worn out.

So, all things considered, I was hoping that a lot of good would come out of this family vacation to California. In addition to having time to reflect and pray about some of the recent events and issues in my life, I was hoping the rest in California would help me regain some of my strength. I was thinking that maybe after two weeks of sightseeing and relaxing in San Diego, Los Angeles, and San Francisco this strange fatigue I had been fighting for months would begin resolving itself and go away.

Where is this Fatigue Coming From?

When I first began noticing I was getting unusually tired, the fatigue was occurring mainly on what is predictably the busiest day of a pastor's week—Sunday.

Our church—Gardendale's First Baptist—is so large and our physical space so cramped that in order for our sanctuary to accommodate our members, we hold three worship services on Sunday mornings. At those three services combined, we average about 3,600 in attendance. I preach at all three services and then at an evening worship service.

Prior to 1999, I didn't feel any significant fatigue on my busy Sundays. Actually, I thrived on all the activity. However, after the fatigue began gripping me, I noticed on Sunday afternoons I was very tired. As that became worse, sometimes on Sunday afternoons I could barely move. I began lying down in the afternoon to get enough strength to do the evening worship service. And I would feel as though my body was literally melting into the bed.

The fatigue began extending from Sundays on into the weekdays. It began affecting my stamina to do exercise. I'm a former high school and college football player, and I've always been physically active. Prior to when I first began experiencing this strange fatigue in 1999, I was swimming a mile a day four or five times a week. To do that mile of swimming at the YMCA pool, I would swim 36 laps and it would take me about 40 minutes a session. However, after the fatigue started bothering me, I had to cut my swimming sessions shorter and shorter. I was saying to myself, "What's going on?" Several weeks before we left for California on that trip, I was already down from 36 laps to 24 laps. By the time we left, I was down even further, to around 18 laps per session. I just couldn't make it any further.

My enjoyable periods relaxing in the YMCA sauna had been cut shorter by my "new tired feeling." I really looked forward to my time in the sauna. I just love to sweat. So I'd go in that sauna and just sweat like crazy for about 30 minutes at a time. But then, after I started getting so tired, I couldn't stand the heat for that long. In the past, I had come out of the sauna feeling invigorated. But then I started coming out feeling drained. I didn't know what the deal was. By the time I went to California, I was down to about 10 minutes per session in the sauna.

I also was experiencing some fatigue during my ministry-related traveling. Since I had been blessed with success in my ministry and was invited to speak around the nation, air travel had become a routine, frequent part of my schedule. Progressively during 1999 and 2000, the fatigue and loss of strength were issues with my travel. One thing I noticed had to do with carrying my briefcase through airports. Since I usually was scheduled to preach and/or teach at my destinations, I would be carrying a briefcase filled with papers and books related to my presentations. In the past, carrying that briefcase had never bothered me. However, after I began feeling weak and tried, I started noticing that I would switch hands with the briefcase. I wouldn't carry it very far before my arm and hand would get tired and I'd have to switch the briefcase to the other side. I thought, "Where is this coming from?"

In addition to taking Sunday afternoon naps and cutting back on the swimming and my time in the sauna, I also took other steps to address the fatigue. I even bought a hammock. On Sunday afternoons, I would get in the hammock and lie there resting for two hours. Then strangely I would get up feeling as tired as when I had first started the rest period. I thought, "What is this? All I'm doing is resting! Something is *wrong!*"

I wracked my brain trying to think of why this was happening to me. Maybe it's just because I'm getting older, I thought. But deep in my mind I knew that at age 42 I wasn't all of a sudden falling apart for no specific reason.

Maybe the trip to California would help.

God's Own Answer

I've been a Christian and a minister long enough to know that God does always answer prayers. I also know that He answers prayers in His way, and on His time schedule. And sometimes God will answer your prayers in a way you least expect and perhaps in a way you don't think you want.

It had been my prayer that the vacation trip to California would somehow help improve my condition by making me more rested.

As it turned out, my symptoms became worse instead of better while we were in California. However, as a result of the symptoms getting worse, this proved to be the first step toward a diagnosis and the treatment I needed.

So the Lord did help me during that trip to California—in His own way.

The Sneeze

Donna and the kids and I were sitting in a movie theatre in San Diego when all of a sudden I sneezed. It was just an ordinary sneeze. Then I blew my nose. What happened to me next was not ordinary at all.

Taken aback by what had just taken place, I turned to my wife in surprise and said, "Donna, my eyes just crossed!"

She said, "What????"

"Yeah. They're crossed," I told her. "I sneezed and blew my nose, and when I blew my nose my eyes crossed."

I left the movie and went to the lobby restroom to see if a mirror would reflect the same thing I was feeling. It did. I was looking into the mirror at a guy who was just as cross-eyed as a kid trying to attract attention by deliberately crossing his eyes. The only thing was, if someone was crossing his eyes on purpose to joke around, he usually could uncross his eyes at will. I could not force my eyes to uncross. I thought, "Man, this is nuts!"

After that happened, my eyes bothered me the whole vacation. I was experiencing double vision, and my left eyelid was drooping. I really fought it and even tried to drive. But it was so bad that when I tried to drive I'd find myself shutting one eye so that I wouldn't be seeing two of everything.

Finally, I decided I had to see a doctor about this even before we returned home. I went to an optometrist in Downey, California. After checking my eyes, he told me, "I don't know what you've got. But it's not your eyes. Your eyes seem fine. When you get back home, you need to see a neurologist."

I knew that a neurologist deals with your brain and spinal cord and nerves and those kinds of things. So I asked the optometrist, "What do you mean, I need to see a neurologist?"

The optometrist replied, "Well, I don't see that this is your eyes. But *something* is wrong with you. You could even have a brain tumor."

To say the least, the optometrist's words got my attention.

On a Fast Track

From the time we arrived home from California, life was on a fast track as it related to my health.

Still thinking that maybe the root of my problem was with my vision, I decided to go first to an ophthalmologist rather than a neurologist.

The Birmingham ophthalmologist confirmed what the optometrist in California had said. He told me, "Son, you've got 20-20 vision in both eyes. The problem is not with your vision. You really do need to see a neurologist."

He referred me immediately to a neurologist in the same building where he had his office. Within 30 minutes, this neurologist, Dr. C. William Barr, III, told me, "You have myasthenia gravis."

I had never heard of myasthenia gravis, also known as MG. In short order, I found out that most of my friends and family members had never heard of it either. There's just not a high level of public awareness about this rare muscle-weakness disease. As soon as some of my friends and family members went to the Internet in search of more information about MG, they became very concerned about me. I particularly recall one minister friend of mine who telephoned me and said, "Steve, man, this myasthenia gravis stuff can be bad!"

Once I had a diagnosis, I was told there was no cure for MG, only treatments for my symptoms. To control the symptoms, I would have to take medications.

It wasn't long before I learned that I also would need additional treatment beyond the medications. Dr. Barr had ordered a bunch of tests done on me—blood work, a CAT scan, and a MRI. And one of those tests, the CAT scan, showed something the medications couldn't take care of.

Donna and I were shopping at a Birmingham department store when we received the news of what the CAT scan had found. My cell phone rang, and it was Dr. Barr's office calling. The CAT scan had shown that I had a tumor on my thymus gland, which occurs in about 10 percent of MG patients. This meant I had to have surgery called a thymectomy to remove my thymus gland. The surgery would be major surgery. In order to reach my thymus gland, the surgical team would have to split open my sternum—my breastbone—just as they do to reach the heart of someone who is having open-heart surgery.

Things were indeed moving fast. I have a vivid memory of how emotional it was for Donna and me when we received that phone call telling us I would have to have surgery. Donna and I both are devout Christians and we're working in a full-time ministry, and we both have a strong faith. But we also are human. When I heard the news that I had to have surgery, and that I had to undergo the surgery right away, I was devastated. I was so overcome that I started crying. Standing there with Donna in that department store, in my mind I just tried to add up all this quickly and put it in perspective. Prior to when that mysterious fatigue had begun creeping into my life about 18 months back, I'd never been sick to amount to anything in my life. Oh, I had suffered a football injury in high school. But I really had never had a major illness. Now everything was suddenly different. I had just learned I was suffering from this strange incurable neuromuscular disease. And I had just been told I had to have major surgery right away.

All of us have lives that include activities that are important to us. When a health problem suddenly interrupts your life, it's easy for your mind to turn not only to your health problem but also to the disruption your health problem is causing in the normalcy of your life. In my case, the timing of all this came when our son, Grant, was about to begin his senior year at Gardendale High School and thus also begin his last season as a high school varsity football player. As Donna and I were leaving the department store that day after learning that I was about to have surgery, I was praying to the Lord just to let me see my son play football.

On August 7, Birmingham surgeon Dr. J. Thomas Williams, Jr. removed my thymus gland. I did well, and the laboratory reports were good. There was no malignancy. I had no post-surgical complications. As an aside, I will report that my doctors told me I had the largest thymus gland they had ever seen. They actually sent reports on it to somewhere in Washington, D.C.

After my surgery, the most difficult thing for me was sitting at home, not being able to preach.

Soon I was back in the pulpit.

And, as it turned out, when Gardendale High School's football season opened a few weeks later, I was in the stands watching and cheering. I attended every game that season, and I videotaped every game. During this period, I still was having double vision. But I was able to watch those ballgames with one eye, and I could videotape the games using one eye.

The first football game of the season was one that drew strong interest in our church. Gardendale High School was playing its archrival, Mortimer Jordan High School. Several members of both of those teams and their families attend our church, and as such we have a friendly high school football rivalry going on in the church.

I was extremely happy that I recuperated fast enough from my surgery that I was able to attend that season-opener game between Gardendale and Mortimer Jordan. In fact, I was so happy that when I got to the game that night I kind of put it way in the back of my mind that I'd just undergone major surgery four weeks previously. From the time we made our way to our seats in the stands, I got caught up with everyone else in the excitement of the game. I was not a recuperating surgical patient. I was a typical football fan and proud dad of a football player out on the field.

Looking back, I tend to smile every time I think of something that happened to me during the game when I got real excited over a play made by our son, Grant. Now, Grant is a big ole boy, very strong. And it's not just the proud dad in me talking when I say that he was a really outstanding football player. We weren't very far into the game when Grant came up with this great play, and, without thinking, I just automatically did what I usually would have done. I turned around to a friend near me and slapped my right hand up to his with enthusiasm to give him a strong "high five." Now, having just had my sternum split open four weeks earlier, that was not the thing for me to do. Man, as soon as I reached up and pushed forward forcefully to give that high five, I started hurting so bad where they had split me open that I thought I was going to die! There was a lady nearby who had a pompom, and I accidentally knocked that pompom about 50 feet as I reacted and cried out in pain, saying, "Ohhh, man. I can't believe I did that!" People started running toward me to help me, yelling out, "Brother Steve, are you okay?" Fortunately,

I had done no lasting damage. I told them, "Yeah, I'm okay. But there will be no more high fives from me during *this* game!"

My View of Today

As I relate this story in March 2002, it has been some 19 months since I stood at that ballgame shortly after learning that I had myasthenia gravis and undergoing a thymectomy.

My life today is full and blessed, in some ways much the same, and in other ways quite different.

Overall, I'm feeling a lot better than I did back in the year 2000. I'm having a great time with my ministry and my life. At the same time, I know that every day I must manage this disease called myasthenia gravis. I do that with the help of medicines and a slower-paced schedule. When I get tired, I just have to sit down. In managing this disease, I *must* get the rest I need.

After I was diagnosed with MG, I went rapidly from never having heard of the disease to finding out a great deal about it. One thing I learned was that this disease creates muscle weakness in MG patients in such a wide variety of ways. Some MG patients have only the eye-related muscle weakness. Other MG patients have muscle weakness in their arms and legs and chewing muscles and other parts of the body, but their eyes are not affected at all. Then there are those who have the same situation that I do, in that they have eye-related problems plus muscle weakness in other parts of the body.

Also, some people have very severe MG situations that even include life-threatening symptoms like weakness of the muscles related to breathing. Others have rather light cases. I fall somewhere in between.

I think I've come to the point of being able to evaluate my own MG situation rather realistically. I have decided that what I have is life-changing and life-altering, but to this point it has not been life-threatening. And it's not overwhelming. It's not something that has to defeat me. I have not come to this view as some kind of "rah-rah cheerleader" but, like I said, just in being realistic.

As part of being realistic, I realized very soon after I was diagnosed that I had to cut back on my very busy schedule if I expected to control the myasthenia gravis. So I cut back. Even before I learned that I had MG, my staff and I already were contemplating a restructuring of our organizational chart. After my diagnosis, we implemented those changes. What the changes mean is that I can continue to function as senior pastor while at the same time delegating much of the day-to-day administrative load that I handled before.

In learning to live my life constructively with MG as a part of it, I've had to make adjustments in both lifestyle and attitude that I know I never could have made without the good Lord as my partner. I have a great and wonderful Lord, and He has been walking with me every step.

I have a great life, and I'm enjoying it more than ever before. There is no doubt that having MG has given me a renewed appreciation of my life, my activities, and everyone in my life. I thought I appreciated all that before. Now I *really* feel appreciation. I don't take much of anything for granted anymore.

Never before have I enjoyed and appreciated my family more than I do today.

Although I've been deeply in love with my wife, Donna, since shortly after I started dating her on December 1, 1978, never have I loved her more than I do today.

I'm taking great pride in watching the growth of our son, Grant. He's in his first year at Union University in Jackson, Tennessee, the same college from which his mother and I both graduated. Grant is studying to become a minister.

We have two cheerleader daughters, ninth-grader Lindsey and seventh-grader Allison. I have a lot of fun attending school ballgames and watching our girls help lead the crowd in cheering for their team.

And our youngest, 8-year-old Bethany, is turning out to be quite a good singer. I've always enjoyed singing and playing the acoustic guitar, so I feel a real fatherly pride there.

I'm relishing every minute of the time I spend with my "church family" and my other friends—just sharing with them, laughing with them. People have been incredibly wonderful to me through all this.

And finally, never before since I first became a pastor at age 25 have I enjoyed my ministry more than I do today. I find this a particularly exciting time to be leading the ministry of our church. We've been able to resolve those problems our church was having back in the year 2000 in procuring land for expansion. In fact, we already have embarked on our $53 million relocation and expansion project.

Although MG impacted me with muscle weakness that affects many parts of my body, I am blessed that thus far I have not been among the MG patients to have weakness of the voice. My voice is as strong as it ever was. And I thank God for the continued strength of my voice when I preach those three services on Sunday mornings, the one on Sunday evenings, and the one on Wednesday nights. I view it as a blessing that in spite of the MG I'm still able to carry on my ministry. It's a blast for me just to drive to work, because I'm still doing what I want to do.

Recalling the Journey

To get to where I am today in living my life with MG, it has been quite a journey. It has been a spiritual journey, a medical journey, and a self-assessment journey.

On the following pages, I want to share bits and pieces of my journey with readers of this book. I do this with the knowledge that many of those reading this book will have a close connection to MG or to some other chronic disease. I hope what I relate in some way touches many of you. In many instances, my goal in sharing something will be to connect with others who have faced a similar challenge. In many instances, all I can do is describe the challenge; I will have no solution to offer; I can only tell you that I have faced this problem and have made peace with it. After years of counseling as part of my ministry, I know that it often can be comforting and inspiring just to know that someone else has faced the same challenge you are facing and still is living a productive life.

In sharing some of my experiences, one thing I want you to know is that even though I have made significant progress during the past two years, I still don't have perfect peace about MG all down pat. I can identify with the struggles faced by all MG patients, and, for that matter, with struggles faced by all patients with various types of chronic diseases.

The Challenge of Prednisone

If I were asked to identify the biggest single "valley" I've traveled in the medical part of my journey, it would have to be my challenges in taking the steroid medication called prednisone. While I know that prednisone has helped me tremendously—and I'm still taking it—I also know it has brought me problems.

One of the side effects experienced by many who take prednisone is weight gain. Boy, have I gained weight! I had never before experienced a weight problem. I'm tall—6 feet, 3 ½ inches. And for the past 20 years I had weighed 230 pounds. But the prednisone really shot me up. I'm now up to about 275 pounds.

To control my muscle-weakness symptoms as much as possible, doctors prescribed both prednisone and a medication known as Mestinon®. My doctors told me that as time went on, there was a chance I could get enough benefit out of having the thymectomy that I could reduce or perhaps even stop taking one or both of these medications. However, until if and when that time came, I would need both the Mestinon® and the prednisone. I needed them to help control the muscle weakness that was making me so weak and exhausted.

The muscle weakness I have experienced with MG has affected different parts of my body. To this day, I tend to experience some or all these symptoms to a greater extent if I over-do and don't get my rest. There are times when my legs are as weak as water. When I'm really tired I will have weakness in my chewing muscles and occasionally in my swallowing muscles. And there are times when I'll have muscle twitching all over my body.

However, there's no doubt that by far my worst MG symptoms have been with my eyes. And those symptoms with my eyes thus far have not allowed me to get off the prednisone.

With my eyes, I've had chronic problems with double vision and drooping eyelids. My eyelids get so lazy that my eyes just won't stay open, particularly the left one. Even after I was diagnosed and went on medication, it took months for the medication to take hold enough to open up both my eyes. While my family and I were on that memorable vacation to California in July 2000, my left eye closed and it didn't open up until four months later, on Thanksgiving Day.

Once the eye did open up, I thought, "This is great! Now I can get off the prednisone and just stay on the Mestinon® and maybe get some of this weight off."

That was not to be, at least not then. After being able to open that eye for about a month and a half, the eye started closing again. When it started closing, I already had started tapering off the prednisone. I had to go back on it. After a few weeks I was able to open the eye again and it stayed open for months. So I tried again to gradually get off the prednisone. This time I cut down gradually until I came totally off of it. And then, while I was attending the Southern Baptist Convention, that left eye closed up again.

When the left eye closed that time, that was the hardest time for me in dealing with the fact I had to take the prednisone. I just thought, "Am I ever going to get off this stuff? Am I ever going to quit gaining weight?" To date, I've tried three times to come off the prednisone and every time the left eye has closed back and I had to start back taking it.

So what have I learned? I think I've learned a few things about controlling vanity. I still would like to lose some weight. However, I have learned that I don't have to look like something out of a *GQ* magazine for God to use me for good.

And, for now, I'm glad both prednisone and Mestinon® are there to help me. I do what my doctor says in taking these medications, at the times and in the dosages the doctor prescribes.

Shedding Stress

I am convinced that although the Lord did not cause me to get MG, He has used this experience to teach me some lessons that have made my life richer.

One of the things the Lord has used this for in my life has to do with handling stress.

Prior to finding out I had MG, I allowed myself to stay under a lot of stress. Really, I would stay uptight much of the time. The ministry is a lot of stress. If you let it, it can become a high-worry, high-risk profession.

However, since I've learned I have MG, I don't let things bother me as they once did. Instead I turn these things over to God through prayer. My prayer life really has picked up.

It's just amazing how many things you can let bother you if you don't give them to God. Too, it's easier to *know* you need to turn to the Lord with things that stress you, and it's easier to *say* you're going to do this, than it is to do it. It sounds so easy to say, "Give the stress to God." From personal experience, I know that it's easier to preach this to others than it is to practice it yourself.

Stress can do terrible things to us. For one thing, I've heard and read that stress has been linked to causing many health problems, and to making many already existing health problems worse—including MG. I know for a fact that when MG finally became a full-blown disease with me, I was under a lot of stress.

After I knew I had MG, it was like God hemmed me up and said, "Okay, what are you going to do with stress? Are you going to let it eat you up, or are you going to give it to Me?"

You don't have to look very far in Biblical scriptures to find encouragement for turning to God for help with your problems. In Philippians 4, verses 6 and 7, Paul is telling us that we should be anxious for nothing but that instead we should turn to God. Psalm 55, verse 22 is clear in its message. That message is to cast your burden upon the Lord, and He will sustain you, that He will never allow the righteous to be shaken. And in 1 Peter 5, verse 7, you can find encouragement to cast your cares upon Him, because He cares for you.

In my office at the church, there's a consistent little path that I walk as I spend time with God in prayer. If I feel an issue pressing on me, if I feel that tension rising, I just turn on the prayer burners.

In every aspect of my life, I can feel an improvement since I really made God my partner in managing stress. I don't dwell on worrying about this disease I have. With all the many issues we're facing with this huge relocation and expansion for the church, I go forward with problem solving without all the anxiety. At home with my children, I enjoy my kids more without so much of the worrying and fretting. Since I'm turning stress and worry over to the Lord, life is more enjoyable and easier to live because things that in the past I looked at as being such a big deal now get ironed out without seeming to be such a big deal at all.

Rearranging Priorities

After I was diagnosed with myasthenia gravis, I had to learn to rearrange the priorities in my life. I've had to slow down a lot. In order to slow down, I had to make decisions about where to spend my time and where not to spend my time. I had to prioritize in a way to make more efficient use out of my active hours, and to schedule more resting hours than in the past so I could manage my MG.

Again, as was true in learning how to manage stress more productively, I believe the Lord has led me in reordering my priorities.

Prior to MG, I was always such a busy person. The more I could get into my schedule, the better I felt about it. I truly believe the Lord has used my MG situation to slow me down. All this has come about kind of like it says in The 23rd Psalm: "He maketh me to lie down in green pastures."

I have implemented some changes that have reduced my workload from around 50 to 60 hours a week down closer to 40 hours a week.

One of the changes that has lightened my schedule has been the restructuring of the way we carry out our church's ministry. Another change came through my decision to cut back on accepting outside speaking engagements, that is, speaking and preaching not directly related to my ministry at Gardendale's First Baptist Church.

In restructuring the way we carry out the church's ministry, it's almost as though God was leading us in that direction even before I knew I had MG. Prior to my diagnosis, I had been discussing with some of our church's other ministerial leaders a possible restructuring that would eliminate having so many people report directly to me. Our church is quite large, and as such we have 100 employees, 20 of whom are pastors with various ministerial responsibilities. After my diagnosis, we implemented that shift in our flow chart that we had discussed. Now our executive pastor, David Jett, reports to me; and others along the line report to David. This just takes a huge administrative load off of me. I now can spend my time giving leadership to the church's primary leaders, staff leaders, ministerial leaders, and lay leaders. And I can spend more time in prayer, studying for my sermons and preaching.

In making the other big change in my schedule, I started declining many of the requests I receive to teach and/or preach in various parts of the nation. Prior to my MG diagnosis, I was frequently accepting invitations to speak and thus was doing quite a lot of traveling. I was glad when people asked me to speak. I felt like I was helping the Kingdom of God to grow. But now I think the Lord wants me to invest most of my time here with my church.

Through all of this, our church has continued to grow. It hasn't missed a beat. Throughout my symptoms that led up to my diagnosis and through my dealing with the MG and the treatments, Gardendale's First Baptist Church has continued to grow and thrive. The church is growing so rapidly that in five out of the last seven years our church has led all churches in the Alabama Baptist Convention with new baptisms, new conversions to Christ. Members of our church have continued their strong support both spiritually and financially. While we don't have a large number of wealthy members in our church, we do have a large percentage of members who tithe, who return 10 percent of their earnings to the Lord's work. For the past several years, we have raised several hundred thousand dollars over our projected annual budget. That is true of the current year, in which we are operating with a $7.2 million budget. As for our $53 million relocation and expansion, we knew we were on our way when we procured a beautiful 130-acre tract of land in a convenient location on Interstate 65, a mile and a half from our present location. Construction starts this year, and we're hoping that by the spring of 2004 we will be occupying the first phase of our project. That first phase will include our new 3,500-seat sanctuary. I'm looking forward to preaching in that new sanctuary!

In the course of rearranging my priorities, I have found out that God doesn't want me to do *everything*. Instead, he wants me to do the *best things*. Too, I've found out there's a difference in doing things right and doing the right thing. I'm supposed to do the right things. Currently in my life my priorities are clear. There are three "right things" I'm supposed to do—spend time with the Lord, be with my family, and pastor this church.

Donna and Me

Through almost 22 years of marriage, Donna and I have been confronting the joys and challenges of life with the help of the Lord. Now we have added another challenge—my battle against myasthenia gravis.

From the time we met as fellow students in a Baptist university, Donna and I have been enriched in our relationship and our lives together by the fact that we share a common faith and belief in God.

Donna was only 12 years old when she was listening to a missionary speak one night and sensed a calling on her life to become a full-time Christian servant.

I was a little older when the calling came to me. I grew up in the First Baptist Church in my hometown, Dyersburg, Tennessee, where my father was a deacon and my mother taught the third grade Sunday School class. However, although I became a church member as a kid, I didn't experience a full conversion until I was 18 years old. After this conversion occurred in a little Tennessee country church, I began sensing a strong desire to talk to people about the Lord—to share my faith with others. At the time, I was pursuing what had been a long-time passion for me—football. I was on full athletic scholarship playing football at a small college, the University of Tennessee at Martin. Prior to suffering a high school football injury (from which I made a great recovery), I had been recruited by larger colleges in the Southeast. Football had been so important to me for so long that I knew a new strong force was at work in my life when football started being less and less important. That started happening immediately after I accepted the Lord at that little Tennessee country church. I just sensed a calling to tell other people about the

Lord; and that was what was on my mind, not football. After I finished my sophomore year, I turned my back on my athletic scholarship and on playing football and headed for a Baptist college, Union University, to answer a calling from the Lord.

Thus, from the time beautiful Donna Dodds and I met at Union University, we were on the same track with the same goals.

Since Donna and I married in 1980, I have pastored three churches and she has been an integral part of the ministry at all three. The first was in Texas, and the second was in Tennessee. And it has been 11 years now that we've been near Birmingham, Alabama, at Gardendale's First Baptist Church.

Donna and I have supported one another in the ministry. We have supported one another as parents. We supported one another in advancing our formal education. After we married, she went on to get her master's degree at Texas Woman's University; and I received both a master's and a Ph.D. from the Southwestern Baptist Theological Seminary in Fort Worth, Texas.

Never has Donna supported me more than since I began battling MG. Her support was there long before I knew what was wrong with me. She was there for me on some memorable Sundays after I had preached three services, and when, as God is my witness, I was so exhausted I didn't know if I was going to make it from the sanctuary to my truck to get home. After I underwent the surgery to remove my thymus gland, Donna was the one sitting there rubbing my feet, bringing me comfort and relief when my feet for some reason just tingled like crazy. My beautiful Donna was the one who was so understanding when I could no longer do yardwork, when I no longer could help her very much around the house, because I had to conserve my limited supply of strength and energy. I'll admit it has been a really humbling experience to realize I no longer have the strength and stamina to do things I had been doing all my adult life. But even at times when I could feel like a lazy bum, Donna never makes me feel like one. She's just there to understand and support. She has stood by me. She's been absolutely wonderful. I *know* that Donna loves me. And I love her.

Donna is physically beautiful. She also is a beautiful person. I'm so crazy about my wife that I will honestly tell you that I'd rather be with Donna than anybody in the world. But no matter how much I loved her before I got myasthenia gravis, I've never loved her more than I do today. I thought I loved her before this; but man, now I *know* I do. I always knew I would do anything for her, but now I *know* I would. Since I got myasthenia gravis Donna and I are more in love than we've ever been.

Through dealing with myasthenia gravis, I've realized how much I not only love my wife but how much I *need* my wife.

Humbling Experience

In responding to Donna's support I've been able to realize how much I need other people as well. Through responding to Donna, it has helped me to open up and be able to accept other people being concerned about me and helping me and doing things for me. I don't take advantage of the caring and compassion others show to me, but I have become open to it.

Having been a minister for so long, having always been so healthy and self-sufficient, I had always been accustomed to helping others rather than others having reason to help me. As an adult, I had never really been dependent on anybody.

After I got MG, it was hard for me at times to accept the help of others. The Lord has helped me with this, through showing me how to be more accepting and humble. I've learned how to swallow some of my pride in terms of allowing others to give me some support. The Lord has helped me to accept support from Donna and our other family and friends. The Lord also has helped me to become more dependent on Him.

Feeling their Concern

As soon as I was diagnosed in the summer of 2000, I shared the news with members of my church. I made my announcement from the pulpit during the morning worship services. At the time, I still didn't understand much about my own condition. But I told them what I knew.

About the initial diagnosis, I said, "I've got a form of whatever this disease is that is called myasthenia gravis." About the thymus gland tumor, I explained, "I've got a tumor the size of a tangerine, and I've got to have it taken out. That means I'll be in the hospital and then home recuperating, so I can't be here with you for a while."

As senior pastor of our church, I feel a special closeness with my church family, and they feel a closeness to me. As I made my announcement, I could hear collective gasps from the audience.

There are not words to describe how supportive and sweet the members of my church have been about all this. I know they always have prayed for me, as I have prayed for them. In recent months, they *really* have prayed for me.

Members of the church family are so tuned in to me that they know when I feel good and they know when I don't. They actually can just look at me and see how things are going. In addition to praying for me, they ask how I'm doing and express their concern. Many of them send me cards and letters. And many have sent or brought food.

I've been through life's peaks and valleys with many of those in the church, through baptisms, weddings, illnesses, funerals, etc. And now they're going through my MG battle with me. For example, there's one little lady in the church who has just started a weekly little ritual of encouragement since I've been diagnosed. She's so nice. I've known her throughout my ministry here. In fact, I officiated at her husband's funeral several years ago. What she does is that at the same time every week she sends me a card of concern and good wishes. She has not missed a single week since I was diagnosed with MG almost two years ago. I receive her card in the mail the same day every week—every Friday.

The Role Models of Edgar and Dorothy

As I live my life now with the reality of myasthenia gravis as a background, I find myself calling on the self-discipline I started learning when I was a child.

My parents, Edgar and Dorothy Gaines, taught my older brother, Ed, and me about focus, self-discipline, and a strong work ethic. They not only taught those things; they practiced those things in their own lives.

When Ed and I were growing up, we had as role models our parents who were confronting life's challenges with their own brand of strength and focus. They were tough as toenails!

My parents did not have the educational opportunities I have been blessed to have. My dad went through the ninth grade, and my mother went through the eleventh grade. Despite a lack of formal education, they just went forward and did what they had to do.

The reason my dad didn't go any further in school is that when he was in the ninth grade his dad got sick. Being the oldest child, my daddy became the man of the house and went to work to make a living for the family.

After serving in the Navy during World War II, my dad returned home and got a job on a railroad. In addition to working for the railroad for 30 years, he also managed our small family farm. My dad was just a quiet, simple, hard-working guy—a railroader, a farmer, and a church deacon. He taught my brother and me to work. And we worked, including chopping coton on our farm.

My mother was somewhat of an entrepreneur. She started a janitorial service. My brother and I were among the some 50 employees who ultimately worked in our mother's janitorial service. One thing I remember well is that the local bank there in Dyersburg, Tennessee, was a client of my mother's janitorial service. When we would be in the bank doing our scrubbing and cleaning, some of these well-dressed bank customers would kind of look down on me because I was holding a mop. I remember what my daddy told me about that. He said, "If you're doing honest work, don't you hold your head down!" That was a real lesson to me that has served me well in the ministry. No matter what station someone might hold in life, that person has value.

I also learned about human kindness and goodness from my parents. Both of them just touched so many people. My mother has been credited with helping to lead a lot of people to Christ in her role as Sunday School teacher to third-grade children. (It's amazing how many preachers came out of that little small-town church!)

The teachings of Edgar and Dorothy Gaines are with me daily as I deal with this MG disease and try to create some kind of reasonable balance with my activities. While on the one hand I know that I must get enough rest to manage my disease, I also know that I can't rest *all the time*. Even if I lie down to rest for a couple of hours, it's not an option for me not to get up and go on and do the things I need to do. I must fulfill my responsibilities. As Edgar and Dorothy's boy, I was just brought up that way.

Passing Along Tips to Chronic Disease Patients

I have seven main tips to share in answer to the question, "What kind of advice would you give to other patients with a similar health problem?"

While the chronic disease I am facing is myasthenia gravis, I think what I have to say in these seven areas has some application with other chronic health problems as well. These are my seven tips:

1. Don't become reclusive. In spite of the fact you have a chronic health problem, it's important that you continue to interact with other people. In fact, *because* you have a health problem you should stay involved with others and not become a recluse. If it's possible, get out and do something with your spouse, do something with your kids, do something with other members of your family or your friends. Don't stay cooped up inside. Go to the mall. Go to ballgames. If your health problems are such that you can't go out, then let others come to you and visit. Depending on what your health issues are, you might have to adjust your thinking to putting up with some symptoms while you're involved with others. If that's what you must do, just do it. In the case of myasthenia gravis patients with eye-related symptoms like mine, you might have to go around with one eye shut, you might find it hard to walk with good balance, and you might find yourself losing depth perception. But nevertheless you must force yourself to get out there and do things. Right after I was diagnosed with MG and underwent my thymectomy surgery, I was still having so much trouble with double vision. But I found out how much fun I could have at ballgames using just one eye at a time!

2. If you get tired, don't be shy about telling people around you that

you have to rest. Now, this might sound somewhat opposite to my first tip about getting out and doing things and staying active. Actually, it *is* the other side of the coin. Managing a chronic disease requires that you maintain a balance—that you rest and take care of yourself, but that you also stay involved with life to the degree that you can be involved. In my case, when I get tired, I just tell my family or whoever else is around, "Guys, I'm out of gas. I've got to go sit down (or lie down) for a while." This is one of the many areas in which my wife, Donna, has been so helpful. If she and I are out with our kids and I say I have to stop and rest, she doesn't make a big deal of it. She just says, "Okay, guys, Dad's tired. Let's stop for a while." Donna knows that when I say, "I'm out of gas," that means I'm out of gas. It does not mean, "I'm *almost* out of gas." It means that I've already pushed myself to the brink. So my message to others dealing with MG or other chronic health problems is this: Don't feel guilty or embarrassed if you have to sit down or lie down. Just do it.

3. **Set realistic goals for your life.** If you find out you have myasthenia gravis or some other major chronic health problem, you need to take inventory of your life and your activities and priorities. Likely you will need to make some changes and some choices. Out of this could come some good. You might find you end up delegating a lot of tasks to others, and totally discarding other tasks you didn't need to be doing at all. The result could be that you do better than ever before in making the most out of your time and energy. I have realized that having MG does not mean that I cannot have a good life. I can have and am having a great life! However, because I have MG, I did feel the need to restructure some things in my life. And I have done that.

4. **Find competent doctors you trust and then do what they tell you to do in managing your disease.** If this means you must take treatments with side effects you don't like, take these treatments if you need them to manage your disease. I had to confront that in the case of prednisone. I don't like to take it. But I know I need it. So I take it. In addition to doing the things your doctor tells you to do to take care of yourself, make sure

you avoid the things the doctor tells you to avoid. I had something that was hard for me to give up after I got MG. That was the hot room at the YMCA. Boy, I really loved sitting in that sauna at the Y and sweating it out in all that heat. That was a great feeling for me. However, after I got myasthenia gravis I learned that this disease is heat-sensitive. The doctor told me I couldn't do that anymore. So I don't do it.

5. On the subject of doctors, I have another thought, too: Don't be hesitant to seek an additional doctor's opinion if you think you could benefit.

6. Enjoy every day, actually every *minute*, of your life. Having a chronic health problem can bring home to you that nothing in life should be taken for granted.

7. Depend on the Lord for support, guidance and strength. I don't say this just because I am a minister of the gospel. I say this because it is proven to me again every day of my life how much the Lord means to me.

Food for Thought for Doctors

During the almost two years since I learned I have myasthenia gravis, several messages for doctors have come to my mind. Some of these have to do with myasthenia gravis in particular. Others have to do with dealing with chronic disease patients.

First are some thoughts I have for doctors in their dealings with myasthenia gravis:

- **I would just urge doctors in general to be more aware of myasthenia gravis and its symptoms.** I know that many doctors never see a case of MG. Even some neurologists see very few MG cases over the course of their entire practice of medicine. Just speaking from a lay view, I really believe there are a lot of people out there who have myasthenia gravis but have not been diagnosed. In fact, I wonder if there aren't quite a number of people who have been wrongly diagnosed with something like chronic fatigue syndrome when in reality they have myasthenia gravis. I've been told that it takes some MG patients years to get a correct MG diagnosis. I've heard of MG sufferers going from doctor to doctor trying to get a diagnosis and the doctors having no idea what's wrong with them. It's my understanding that the easiest-to-diagnose MG patients are those who have the eye-related symptoms like I experience. It seems those eye-related symptoms like double vision and drooping eyelids can be a big tip-off to a doctor that someone has MG. But doctors need also to be on the lookout for patients who have MG but who don't have the eye-related symptoms. Looking back to my childhood, I can't help but wonder if my dad's aunt had an undiagnosed case of myasthenia gravis. I don't recall that she had eye-related symptoms, but she had this strange weakness all over her body, this chronic fatigue. She died when I was real young. Back then—35 to 40 years ago—most doctors probably would have known very little about myasthenia gravis. On top of that, this aunt lived out in the country where there was practically no medical care available. But she just had this general overall fatigue that no one in the family could really understand, and it kept her in bed most of the time. I can remember going to see her and asking her family, "Why is she in bed all the time?" The family members told me something to the effect of, "Well, it's hard for her to stay out of bed. She's so weak she can hardly walk. She's just always real tired." Looking back, I can't help but wonder.

• **This is more of a question to doctors than a suggestion: Are there strong tendencies for many MG patients to have a family history of neurological problems?** I ask this because I have heard of family neurological-disease history with some MG patients. Also, here I am with this neuromuscular disease, and my own father suffered from three neurological problems at various times in his life. My daddy had Parkinson's disease, Alzheimer's disease, and Shy-Drager syndrome, a nervous system disorder associated with fluctuations in blood pressure and dizziness and blackouts.

In addition, I have some thoughts for doctors treating all types of chronic diseases.

- **Treat each patient with respect and give that patient your undivided attention while you are with the patient.** I have been fortunate to have doctors who have done this with me, and I can tell you it means everything in the world. It's so important in helping you manage your chronic disease to have a doctor who's in there with you showing a little compassion, a little sincere attention, and practicing the Golden Rule of treating you like he would like to be treated.

- **If your patient seeks another opinion from another doctor, do not make that patient uncomfortable and do not turn your back on that patient.** When you're treating a patient who has to deal with a chronic illness, as a doctor it's time to check your ego at the door.

- **Listen to what your patients tell you.** I have several doctors who are members of my church. I've had some of them tell me that when they listen closely to their patients, it helps the patients and it also helps them to be better doctors. The doctors say that by listening to their patients they become more informed because they learn about the patients' diseases. It's one thing for a doctor to study the books to learn about a disease; but it's a great next step to be able to learn from someone who actually has the disease. A doctor also needs to listen well in order to know how to provide treatment for his (or her) patient.

Some Spiritual Truths

During the spiritual part of my journey since I was diagnosed with myasthenia gravis, I have reaffirmed old spiritual truths, and I have discovered new ones.

In my Thanksgiving 2000 sermon, which I delivered four months after my MG diagnosis, I shared with my church members seven of those truths that really had come home to me. I want to share them with you now:

- God is with us at all times.
- God uses people to minister to us.

- God is manifested in our weakness.
- God comforts us so that we can comfort other people.
- God always answers prayer.
- God, family, and church family are the most important things in our lives.
- Always be thankful, because somebody is worse off than you.

A Newfound Strength

I want to share with you one lesson that has come home to me above all others during my MG experience. It has to do with the meaning of true strength.

Prior to having MG, I think I had become so self-sufficient, and, yes, so self-confident, that at times in one way or another I was saying, "That's okay, God, I don't need You. I can handle this." However, after I got MG, I found myself dealing with something that I *knew* I could not handle on my own.

As I turned to the Lord for help, I could feel the Lord's strength kicking in. Out of this, I was discovering a newfound strength.

Part of this newfound strength was an inner discovery. It was a redefining of what constituted real strength in my life. I began to strip away some of those ideas I had had in the past about what I should be like in order to be strong.

I began to discover that I can function and be a strong person without having all those things together that I once thought I had to have. The weight gain I have experienced as a side effect of taking the prednisone has been a humbling example. Like I said before, now I know I don't have to look like something out of a *GQ* magazine for God to use me. Likewise, I don't have to possess the physical strength to bench-press 300 pounds. I don't have to be able to swim a mile. I don't have to have my financial investments in perfect order as far as I can see into the future. To be strong and effective, I don't have to be able to travel all over the country speaking and preaching all the time. And I don't have to possess the stamina to work 50 or 60 hours a week.

I think it took something startling like MG to show me that I've spent so much of my life swimming upstream, fighting to be successful and handling all too much on my own.

In the midst of the grave physical weakness that myasthenia gravis has brought to the muscles of my body, I have turned to God for support. And in so doing I have found more *inner strength* than I've ever had at any time in my life.

Epilogue

This book was written as a book of information and also as a book of hope and inspiration.

It is my fervent desire that each of you who reads the book will come away with your mind and heart filled with ideas and plans to address the needs of individuals with chronic diseases.

If you are a patient waging a battle against a chronic disease, my wish for you is that the book will inform and motivate you to take actions to improve your own situation.

If you are the family member, friend, caregiver, employer, or other contact of a chronic disease patient, my goal is that you will take away an increased understanding of what the chronic disease patient faces. After you have read this book, I challenge you to help at least one chronic disease patient in a way you have not done previously.

If you are a physician or other healthcare professional who participates in the care of chronic disease patients, I encourage you to look inside yourself for your own ideas and solutions for improving the healthcare of chronic disease patients. And, once you have identified some solutions, put them to work.

If you are a person who has a desire to help chronically ill people in your area, I advise you to light a fire with other citizens in your community and get something going.

If you have reason to learn more about the chronic neuromuscular, autoimmune disease known as myasthenia gravis, I hope you have accepted my invitation to use this book to become familiar with this disease. In the book, I have in many ways used myasthenia gravis as a kind of "representative" for all chronic diseases. I hope that becoming more informed about MG will motivate you to learn more about other chronic diseases as well.

And, finally, if you are in a position to provide philanthropic funds to make inroads into some of these problems involving chronic disease,

I urge you to do so. Through the new foundation I'm establishing, we will be contacting many of you to enlist your funding assistance for our research and patient support programs related to myasthenia gravis and other chronic autoimmune diseases.

This book was written not just to lay out the problems associated with myasthenia gravis and other chronic diseases. It also was written to focus on solutions that already exist and to plant the seeds for new solutions. It was written to rally and rouse those who care and who can help.

I appeal to you, the reader of this book, to look closely at yourself, and ask, "What can I do to help in the battle against myasthenia gravis and other chronic diseases?" After you identify what you can do, waste no time in doing it.

Ronald E. Henderson, M.D.

Index

ABOUT THE AUTHOR

RONALD E. HENDERSON, M.D., has been a medical leader and an entrepreneur for three and a half decades. He was the founder and long-term CEO of Henderson & Walton Women's Center in Birmingham, Alabama, one of the largest freestanding obstetrics and gynecology (OB-GYN) practices of its type in the nation. Dr. Henderson served as a medical leader at the county, state, and national levels. As a member of the governing board for Alabama's public health system, he was instrumental in reorganizing the Alabama Department of Public Health. He was a cofounder of a professional liability insurance company (ProAssurance on the New York Stock Exchange) and a cofounder of one of the first freestanding surgery centers in the Southeast (Birmingham Surgical Center). In 1985, he founded a health maintenance organization; and, in 1992, he founded a physician practice management company. Forced to retire from his medical practice in 1994 due to symptoms of myasthenia gravis (MG), Dr. Henderson was inactive for several years. Now that he has regained his health, he devotes the majority of his time to the battle against MG and other autoimmune diseases. He serves as president of the Alabama Chapter of the Myasthenia Gravis Foundation of America, Inc. Recently, he has established the International Autoimmune Disease Research Foundation that will focus on research in MG and other autoimmune diseases. Dr. Henderson and his wife, Beth, maintain homes in Birmingham and Prattville, Alabama. They have three children and four grandchildren.